Stories for the
Third Ear

Stories for the Third Ear

Lee Wallas

W · W · NORTON & COMPANY
New York   London

Published simultaneously in Canada by Penguin Books Canada Ltd, 2801 John Street, Markham, Ontario L3R 1B4
Printed in the United States of America.

Library of Congress Cataloging in Publication Data

Wallas, Lee.
  Stories for the third ear.

  "A Norton professional book."
  1. Storytelling—Therapeutic use. 2. Hypnotism—
Therapeutic use. 3. Psychotherapy. I. Title.
RC489.S74W35   1985   616.89′16   85-7294

ISBN 0-393-70019-4

W. W. Norton & Company, Inc., 500 Fifth Avenue, New York, N.Y. 10110
W. W. Norton & Company Ltd., 37 Great Russell Street, London WC1B 3NU

This book is dedicated to:

My daughter, Eugenie Wallas Nakell, patient transcriber of tapes, stoic typist of miles of corrections, revisions, and revisions of revisions, my unflagging supporter;

My son, Charles Wallas, unconditional positive regarder;

My grandchildren, David, Adam, and Rebecca Wallas, and Sarah Wallas Powell, intermittent guinea pigs, and claque;

All my friends and colleagues who encouraged me when I faltered;

And above all, my clients through the years who listened with the "third ear" and made this book happen.

Foreword

Milton H. Erickson, one of the most effective and innovative psychotherapists of our time, died on March 25, 1980. Since that time there has been an outpouring of books attempting to transmit and explain his teachings. Erickson stated that "the practice of psychotherapy should be interesting, appealing and charming," and one of the elements in his therapy, particularly in his later years, was the utilization of what I have called "teaching tales." Lee Wallas calls them "stories for the third ear." These stories not only add an element of charm and beauty to the psychotherapy in which they are used, but there is increasing clinical evidence that their use adds to the effectiveness of therapy.

As interpreters of Milton Erickson have pointed out, and as Erickson himself stated, the central elements in his therapy were, "First you model the patient's world; then you role model the patient's world." Both the modeling and role-modeling can be done in the form of stories. The first part of the story analogues the patient's symptoms, problems or life situation, thereby modeling the patient's world, or part of it. The second part of the story analogues or role-models solutions or optional ways of looking at or dealing with the patient's situation.

The excellent stories presented here by Lee Wallas, who is a creative and experienced therapist, follow this Ericksonian prescription. And, as Erickson said of some of his own tales, the stories "came to her" when she herself was in a trance state. They were presented to patients who were also in a trance state.

Erickson defined hypnosis as "the evocation and utilization of unconscious learnings." He felt that we are in closest touch with our own inner knowledge and in best rapport with our patients or clients when both of us are in a "shared" trance. He believed that we are most open to learning in that state. Lee Wallas gives therapists clear and explicit directions for helping patients to enter and utilize these "learning trances." She also shares with us some of her ways of preparing them to "receive the riches." The Sufis and others felt that this preparation was most important in the imparting of any teaching.

Simply entering into a trance state seems to enable most therapists to tap the poetic elements of their own psyche and it may be that this poetic element is directly connected with emergence of "unconscious" mentation, hopefully of a wise nature. Of course, Wallas does not imply that the mere telling of a tale will cure anyone. She describes many other therapeutic factors (e.g., insisting that an alcoholic patient attend A.A. meetings), often involving months or even years of work. But one cannot help but be impressed by the power of a teaching tale, when it is utilized properly. I have seen and heard of many instances in which patients' behavior has changed positively after a teaching tale has been utilized—either one which was borrowed from Erickson, from the Bible, from folk tales, or one which was created by the therapist.

Experienced therapists will certainly find that studying the composition and use of language in Lee Wallas' stories can inspire them and help them to develop their own "teaching tales." These tales need not be in the form of fairy tales. They could just as easily evolve around science fiction, poetry, other literary forms, even recipes or menus. They might involve the use of music or movement metaphors, as expressed in dance.

Therapists who explore these approaches will be moving in directions which Erickson encouraged—towards the discovery of more effective ways of helping people to "learn to think" and to grow.

Sidney Rosen, M.D.
Founding President
New York Milton A. Erickson
Society for Psychotherapy and Hypnosis

Prologue: The Three Lessons

Once upon a time, there lived a witch. She was very, very old. She was also very wise because she had lived such a long time, and had so many experiences. She had experienced many things, many, many things. Now this particular witch practiced an interesting kind of magic, a special kind of magic, so that people far and wide heard about her magic and would come to her to learn.

One day, a young woman knocked on her door. The witch opened the door wide and asked, "What are you seeking?" And the young woman answered, "I want to learn everything that you know so that I can be as wise as you and become a witch like you and practice magic like you." The witch looked deep into her eyes and saw there that the young woman knew everything she needed to know except that she didn't know that she knew. And so the witch said, "Please come in." And that was the first lesson.

Then she said, "I cannot teach you in words alone." That was the second lesson. Then she said, "Time is very short, so you must always give your complete attention." And that was the third lesson.

Then the witch said, "Now you are ready for knowing." The young woman laughed with delight and eagerly held out her open hands. The old witch smiled, nodded with approval, and said, "Yes." The lessons were over and the young woman continued her journey.

Contents

Contents

Stories for the Third Ear

Introduction

Nietzsche, in *Beyond Good and Evil,* used the phrase "the third ear," meaning that it is with the "third ear" we hear the metaphorical language of our intuition.* We dream in metaphor, and at our deepest levels we dialogue in metaphor, and through metaphor we can achieve fundamental understanding.

Milton Erickson, that great genius of hypnotherapy, used anecdote as metaphor to effect what often seemed to be miraculous cures. His innovative use of storytelling has opened up limitless possibilities for effective psychotherapy. The anecdotes that Erickson told were gathered throughout his rich life experience, and they most admirably suited his style. Unlike his, my stories are not anecdotal. Rather, they are imaginary fables that have presented themselves spontaneously from time to time. I do not plan for them, and I never know in advance when they will "tell themselves." Nor do I know in advance how they will develop or conclude. I do know that they come directly from my unconscious, and that they are addressed to my client's "third ear." They usually occur when

*Nietzsche, Friedrich. *Beyond Good and Evil.* Chapter VIII, section 246, pp. 180-1. New York: Carlton House.

my client is in a state of somnambulistic trance, and I myself am in a somewhat altered state of consciousness. The language of my unconscious proves to be quite child-like, which is, I believe, an important component of the therapeutic effectiveness of these particular stories. Once I had a fine teacher who said, "If you want to be heard when you teach, then speak as if addressing an eight-year-old."

Although I never consciously plan when a story will "tell itself," I am aware that in every instance the story arrives only after I have established a trusting relationship with my client. Apparently the story is formulated in my unconscious only after I have reached a clear understanding of the client's frames of reference, principal representational field, vocabulary, perception of his problems, and feelings about himself and his situation.

I have chosen to include these particular stories because in each case the story proved to be a turning point in the course of treatment. Significant change and improvement seemed to stem from that time. Certainly this is not surprising when we recall that storytelling has been the vehicle for teaching since earliest history. Stories are the roots of all history as we know it, the oldest form of exchanging human knowledge and experience. In many simple cultures, even in our own time, storytelling is a very important aspect of the socialization process. It introduces and reinforces cultural values. In our more complex culture, the stories children tell and hear serve the same purpose.

I recall that when I was a little child, no more than six years old, I discovered the Cabanne Branch Library within roller-skating distance from my house. My life was transformed! Every afternoon after school, I would skate there. I had discovered stories, and *all of them were about me*! I began to live the rich and varied lives of fairy tale princesses, Indian maidens, Greek goddesses, and countless others. I encountered overwhelming problems, and I learned how to overcome them. Every day brought a new triumph. Of course, the stories I read were metaphors for my own experiences. I translated the conflicts into those I met in my daily life, and the characters were transformed into the real people I actually knew. Surely, the boy next door never realized that he was really Attila the Hun.

Milton Erickson structured his anecdotes so that they were analogous to the life situations of his patients. His metaphors included familiar details supplied by the client's frame of reference. For example, in the well-known case of Joe, a florist intensely interested in plants who was suffering great pain from terminal cancer, Erickson talked about the cycle of the tomato.* Naturally, this subject engaged Joe's interest without arousing his resistance.

It is exactly in this way that stories "work" with my clients. They bring the story into the framework of their own experience. They try to make sense of it as it would apply to them. And although the content of the story is a metaphor which evokes but does not literally reproduce the actual circumstances of clients' lives, they can accept what the story seems to imply about their problems and consider new solutions within the framework of their own lives.

I agree with those who perceive the unconscious to be protective. Before we can let go of our dysfunctional behavior, the unconscious needs to be persuaded that we can safely choose other options which will work better for us and be more gratifying to us. Establishing rapport and lowering resistance open the door for the unconscious to translate the

---

*Erickson, M. H. *The Collected Papers of Milton H. Erickson on Hypnosis. Volume IV: Innovative Hypnotherapy.* Ernest L. Rossi (Ed.). New York: Irvington, 1980, pp. 268-275.

metaphor of a story and incorporate new possibilities. How do we establish such a trusting relationship? I would like to describe one way to prepare clients for hypnotherapy, which has proven to be the most successful way for me. Unlike Erickson, I never start treatment with stories. Lacking his phenomenal skills, experience, and reputation, I need more time to establish rapport. My first step, like his, is to hear the client's story, noting vocabulary, body language, frames of reference, representational fields, as well as story content, and his problems as he perceives them. I also want to know about the other significant characters that people his life. While all this is taking place, I assume, as closely as possible, the client's physical posture and his breathing rhythm. I also do a lot of affirmative head-nodding and "uh-huhs." At the end of the first session I say, briefly, that he must feel most uncomfortable (or unhappy, sad, angry, frustrated, stuck) and that I am glad he came in for treatment.

In the second session we review the client's story briefly and talk about any new occurrences between sessions. Then I ask him what myths and suppositions he has heard about hypnosis before coming for treatment. I then answer any questions that he may have about the methods of hypnotherapy and explain in general what happens, emphasizing that the client is always in charge, that his unconscious protects him and will bring him directly out of trance should he feel threatened in any way. I assure him that no one can persuade him in trance to do or think anything which is not in his own best interest or would not be acceptable to him in full consciousness. As an example of the protective role of the unconscious, I say that he has probably experienced sleeping soundly at night undisturbed by accustomed noises. Garbage trucks can grind and squeal at 4 a.m., cans can bang, cats can wail, and he sleeps on peacefully. However, let the slightest unusual noise occur—a window raised or a stair tread creaking—and he is instantly wide awake and alert. It is his "protective witness" guarding his safety. The unconscious never sleeps and never relaxes its vigilance. I wind up this session by telling him that I plan to make a tape recording for him during our next session and that I will explain the purpose of the tape at that time.

The third session begins like the first sessions with a brief recap designed to reassure the client and to strengthen rapport. When the client appears to be at ease, I explain that I will use this session to make a tape especially for him. I add that I will explain its use and purpose when we have completed the tape, at which time he can decide if he wants to make use of it. I take great care consistently to give him the power of decision.

In my office I have a bed-sized couch. I ask the client to remove his shoes, generally make his clothing loose and comfortable, and then lie down and pretend that he is going to bed for the night. I mention that it is okay to fall asleep, that we hear very well when we are asleep. Perhaps we incorporate what we hear even better than when awake. I ask if he has ever heard that one can learn a foreign language by listening to records while sleeping, and then I affirm that it is true. I begin recording, after suggesting that it would be better for him not to speak until I have finished since he will not want to hear his own voice on the tape. I always start out with the same message, adding only minor variations for particular needs:

"Lie down in your bed, relax, let the bed hold you up. Let go . . . and then let go again . . . and again. Concentrate on your breathing. Pretend there is a balloon right under your belly button. When you breathe in, the balloon fills WAY UP with air; when you breathe out, the balloon collapses almost all the way down to your spine. That is the natural way to breathe. That is the way babies and puppy dogs breathe. The natural way to breathe fills your lungs with good pure oxygen all the way to the very bottom, and expels the carbon dioxide and other poisons all the way from the very bottom on out of your body. Just breathe slowly and naturally."

This technique is derived from Yogic breathing exercises, and I use it repetitively in subsequent sessions of trance induction. It is my first step in teaching concentration. I then proceed with detailed instruction, starting with the feet:

"Pay attention to your feet." (My voice has become cadenced with his breathing.) "Relax your heels; relax your insteps; relax the balls of your feet; relax each toe in turn; wiggle your toes a little; let go. Make your feet heavier and heavier." (With obese clients I substitute words like "limp" or "weightless.")

I proceed in this detailed way up the body to the lower legs, the knees, the thighs, the pelvis, the genitals, the buttocks, the abdomen, the small of the back, the torso, the collarbone, the shoulders, upper arms, elbows, forearms, wrists, hands, thumbs, each finger in turn, saying, "Let go . . . and let go again." All of this is delivered in an even, monotonous, quiet tone in rhythm with the client's breathing.

(One of the variations I have used to adapt this deep relaxation exercise to particular needs is an added injunction which emphasizes some special condition. For example, in treating a client with multiple sclerosis whose right hand had become rigid and immobilized, I added, "You might relax the muscles in your right hand . . . and relax them again. Compare the relaxed feeling in your left hand with the relaxed feeling in your right . . . let go . . . now move the fingers of your left hand and visualize in your mind's eye how you did that. Now visualize the fingers of your right hand moving in just that same way. Now if you wish you can WIGGLE THE FINGERS OF

YOUR RIGHT HAND a little." *Mirabile dictu!* She succeeded in doing it. I have read how Erickson taught himself to move again, muscle by muscle, after he was wholly paralyzed by polio, by recalling in painstaking detail exactly how he had moved before his illness. So I knew it was possible for my client to learn to move her paralyzed muscles. In similar ways, I vary the tape to focus on any special needs of each client.)

I continue the tape with suggestions to relax the back of the neck, the scalp, the forehead, the eyelids (at which point many clients are in trance), the cheekbones, the jaw, the chin, the upper lip, the lower lip, the tongue. I conclude this part of the tape with, "Take your mind to any part of your body where you still feel tension . . . and deliberately let go . . . again . . . and again."

Since the first part of the tape is designed to release tension and stress, one of the valuable side effects is the relief of insomnia after hearing the tape each night for a month or so. Other benefits are the clinically demonstrable lowering of high blood pressure and the acceleration of healing. Of course, the primary purpose is to teach the client to focus his or her attention, the first step in trance induction. The soothing, supportive cadence and the hypnotic rhythm of my speech induce tranquility and the release of tension. Throughout the tape there is the inference of being taken care of, of being supported, of being cradled, which produces quiet pleasure and trust. At this point all but the most fearful or angry have become blissfully peaceful and relaxed.

In the second part of the tape, I talk about the great power at the command of our bodies and our minds: "Pay attention to your mind. You have a wonderful brain. In it are stored millions upon millions of facts that you have gathered through the years, even before you were born . . . all there for you, carefully catalogued and available at an instant's notice, more efficient than the most sophisticated computer . . . a treasure store of resources . . . all there for you. You can summon even the most diverse facts at will, sort them out to form options, choose among your options to make decisions, and use your decisions to solve your problems. You can use your fine brain to solve your job problems, your family problems, your relationship problems, your love problems, your money problems . . . any problems you might have. Your brain is your problem-solving instrument. Use it to solve your problems. Don't ask your body to solve your problems. It doesn't know how. Your body knows how to perform at maximum efficiency, to keep itself well, and to heal itself when needed. It doesn't know how to solve your love problems, your money problems" (etc., etc., depending on each client's frame of reference). "Solve your problems with your fine brain and give your body permission to do what it knows how to do."

For a client with heart dysfunction or hypertension, I go into detail. For example, "Pay attention to your heart. Notice how steadily, faithfully it beats, slow, strong, steady, never stopping day or night, waking or sleeping, faithfully pumping the rich, life-giving blood throughout your system, and it has done so since before you were born. It knows how to perform efficiently, to keep itself well, and to mend itself if need be. Don't ask it to solve your problems; it doesn't know how. Solve your problems with your fine brain and give your heart permission to do what it knows how to do."

For respiratory dysfunctions, I translate the same message as it applies to bringing clean oxygen into the lungs and expelling poisons and pollutants, with the added message to smokers: "Your lungs are the sole avenue for bringing life-essential pure oxygen to your bloodstream. Cigarette smoke poisons the oxygen you supply to your body, etc., etc." In this way it is possible to specifically emphasize whatever physical problems are peculiar to each client. I wind up this part of the tape by talking about the powers of the body to heal itself. (The majority of my clients have been "visual" people, thinking and dreaming in pictures and using visual language like, "I see, I perceive, I notice, etc." Occasionally when a client proves to be principally auditory or kinesthetic, I prepare him for the next part of the tape, which is a healing exercise entailing visualization, by *overlapping*.*

I continue the tape with, "Your body has great power to heal itself. Pretend that you are making yourself very small and going down inside your body. Now, take your time and look around carefully until you have spotted the place or places that need healing. (If there is an ongoing dysfunction like ulcerative colitis or asthma, I will specifically mention it.) Now, send out a loud call to your white corpuscles, your white healers. They will come running by the thousands at your command, leaving thousands more back at their usual stations where they continue to guard your well-being. When they have formed a large circle around you, you will see how strong, how powerful, how eager they are to serve you. Perhaps you see them as white soldiers, or perhaps as nurses, or maybe white knights in armor. Some people see them as large white animals. Let yourself see your white healers. . . . Now, send

---

*Overlapping is a technique whereby a client is led from his principal representational field into accepting another representational field. For example, with an "auditory" client, I might say, "Imagine you are listening to music and suddenly, at your door, there is a tremendously loud explosion of noise. Now think of cartoons in a comic book and how a loud noise is indicated. Often it is a picture of a big jagged red circle with the word BANG written across it. Now, imagine the loud noise again, and imagine the comic book with the big red circle with BANG on it." We have overlapped from the heard sound to the seen picture. I do not incorporate overlapping in the tape. Rather, I spend some time beforehand to prepare the client for visualization, a very powerful tool for healing.

out a second loud call to your red healers, your red corpuscles. They, too, come running by the thousands bringing supplies and reinforcements, and they, too, leave thousands more just like them at their regular stations to guard your health.* When the red healers have gathered in a circle around the white healers, you instruct them to go to work. You point out the place or places to them." (Instructions vary depending on the type of dysfunction. In case of infection, perhaps they can see the "germs" as little ugly devils that are easily killed by the powerful "healers." In case of impairment, healing may require soothing, mending, and healing instructions, etc.) "Now, instruct them to stay at their work continuously, without stopping, day and night, waking or sleeping, until you are completely healed, and then, and only then, may they return to their regular stations. When you see that they are hard at work,

---

*I always make sure to mention both white and red "healers" since an incident which occurred early in my practice of hypnotherapy. A client, whom I shall call "Christine," a young woman in her mid-twenties, had been coming to see me because she was experiencing feelings of great anxiety. Late one night I received a call from Christine's husband telling me that she had been hurt in an automobile accident and was hospitalized. Christine urgently wanted to see me. Would I go to the hospital in the morning? When I arrived there Christine complained of a "terrible" pain in her side, and was certain she had suffered a bad internal injury, although her doctor could not find evidence of this. She was quite agitated, saying she did not trust either her doctor or the hospital staff. She asked me to hypnotize her to help her heal herself. I complied, and when she was in a deep trance, I suggested that she summon her white healers to the place inside which needed healing. When she came out of trance she said she felt much better. The next morning she called me, greatly agitated because her white blood count had risen alarmingly high. I then remembered that, in my zeal, I had omitted calling her red "healers"! I returned to the hospital as fast as I could, induced trance, and called both white and red healers. This time I also remembered to mention leaving thousands of red and white healers at their accustomed stations to guard her well-being. Happily, her blood count normalized later that day. And you can believe me that I have never repeated that mistake again!

you come out from inside your body, assured that your healers are all working and will be doing their job until you are healed." This concludes the second part of the tape.

The third part has to do with self-esteem. I begin by saying, "I am going to take you to a very beautiful place. Perhaps it will be a place you remember, where you particularly liked to be. Or, perhaps it will be a place where you long to go. Or, perhaps it will be a place you have imagined. Now you are there . . . you look all about you, taking your time . . . overlooking nothing. You see details vividly — the beautiful colors, and shapes, and lights and darks, enjoying the beauty. . . . Now you look down at yourself and see that you, too, are beautiful. Welcome to the world of beautiful sights. You, too, belong here. Take your place in the world of beautiful sights. . . . Welcome to the world.

"Listen to the sounds you are hearing . . . enjoy each sound in turn. . . . Now listen to your heartbeat, and the rhythm of your own breathing. . . . You, too, make beautiful sounds. . . . Welcome to the world of beautiful sounds. Take your place in it. You belong here in the world of beautiful sounds. Welcome to the world.

"Feel what surrounds you. . . . Perhaps the sun is warm on your skin. . . . I don't know, but you do. Perhaps the feel of cool clear water. . . . Be aware of feeling. . . . Take your time. . . . Now, feel your own smooth body. Run your hands down your own smooth body, and feel how good you are to the touch. Welcome to the world of touching and feeling. You belong here. Take your place in it. Welcome to the world.

"Now, be aware of the smells and fragrances around you. Notice them one by one. Enjoy identifying them. Smell your own healthy odor. . . . Welcome to the world of fragrance and odors. Welcome to the world. You belong here. Take your place in it. Welcome to the world.

"And now . . . you turn, and you notice a large banquet table. It is covered with an elegant embroidered banquet cloth, and on it are gleaming silver, sparkling crystal, and shining china. There are platter on platter on platter of all your favorite foods, and there are pitchers, and carafes of all your favorite beverages. . . . Now you approach and begin to select, first this delicacy and then that . . . taking your time. . . . You sip, first this drink and then that . . . taking your time, chewing slowly, paying attention to flavor . . . and texture before you swallow and feel it settle comfortably in your stomach. You continue, asking yourself from time to time if you are still hungry or if you have had enough. . . . If you pay attention, your stomach will tell you when you have had enough. . . . When your stomach tells you that you have had enough, you will turn away happily, knowing you may return whenever you feel hungry or thirsty. . . . It is all there for you. . . . Welcome to the world of tasting, eating, and drinking. . . . You belong here, take your place in it. . . . Welcome to the world.

"And now you begin a slow, graceful dance. You glide, and you sway, you reach and you kneel, you turn, and you skip, and your dance begins to grow faster and faster until you are leaping and whirling in an exhilaration of movement and vitality. You enjoy your grace and vigor. Welcome to the world of movement and dance. You belong here. Take your place in the world of movement and dance. Welcome to the world. . . . You belong here just like the flowers, and the birds, the sky, and the earth, the sun, the moon, the stars, and the clouds, the trees and the water. You, too, belong here. Welcome to the world. . . . Welcome to the world."

After a pause, I say, "In a little while I shall count to three. If this be daytime, when you hear the count of three, you might stretch, yawn, and at your own pace, taking your time,

you will sit up, and when you . . . OPEN YOUR EYES* . . .
you will feel relaxed, rested, full of well-being . . . you will feel
energized, looking forward eagerly to whatever you have
planned for the rest of the day. . . . If this be nighttime, when
you hear "three," you can reach over, flip off your tape recorder, snuggle under the covers, and fall into a deep restful
sleep. You can awaken at the time you have set for yourself,
and when you awaken you might stretch, perhaps yawn, and
taking your time, at your own pace, you sit up. When you open
your eyes you will feel wonderfully rested and relaxed, full of
well-being and vitality. You can look forward to making your
day the most creative, productive, and enjoyable in your life
so far. . . . One . . . two . . . three." This concludes the tape.

When the client has listened to the tape every night for a
while, commonly there is a marked decrease in tension and
a marked increase in rapport between us. Our work together
is enhanced and accelerated. Also, the sound of my voice often
becomes a cue for the client to go into trance. In the following sessions, I induce trance, aiming for enhanced imagery
and for deeper trance states. In the sense that I use it, imagery
includes more than visualization. The tape includes all the
senses: smell, taste, sight, hearing, and kinesthetic feeling. I
include emotional feelings as well. I am careful not to be
specifically descriptive, because the images a client summons
from within himself or herself are the most powerful. They
are assembled from personal experience, memories, fantasies,
and hopes. I might say, "Go to a favorite place," but I do not
name a place or specify what will be encountered there. Erick-

---

*An embedded message incorporated in a sentence and annotated by an
increase in volume and a slight pause before and after, which I often use
to bring a client out of trance.

son used such phrases as, "Perhaps you will, you might, possibly," etc. His avoidance of direct command opened up possibilities for his patient, tapped the patient's own resources, and sidestepped possible resistance.

Sooner or later, in the course of treatment, a story begins to "tell itself." Most often, there seems to be no significant reaction to the story in that session. Delayed reaction more frequently occurs. Sometimes as many as two or three sessions take place before the client comments on the story or alludes to some part of it.* Sometimes it is never mentioned at all. But what is first noticeable is an evident change, a new plan, a new attitude, or an aura of hopefulness and new resolve. From that point until termination, we work to implement and reinforce the changes.

In conclusion, I would like to summarize what I believe to be the essential ingredients for the effective use of storytelling. First of all, I make careful, thoughtful preparations to establish rapport, before I begin actual storytelling. I believe that rapport, however we establish it, is the magic "open sesame" for the effective use of metaphor. Rapport makes the metaphor available to the client. In turn, the metaphor is powerful because it defuses resistance, in that a story is "once removed" so that the new possibilities it offers become intriguing suggestions rather than commands.

Secondly, the stories in this book are spoken words. They are for reading aloud. Actually, they are transcripts of tapes

---

*Sometimes their reactions are startling, to say the least. I remember one incident after telling a story to a borderline schizophrenic. At the outset of the next session, she opened with, "You know, you are a lot like Jesus." I thought, "Jesus! Oh, no, now she has added religious delusion to her repertoire." I asked in what way did she see me as resembling Jesus. She replied, "Well, in the Bible Jesus taught his followers by telling stories, and that is what you do." I breathed a long sigh of relief.

recorded during the treatment sessions. They begin spontaneously without previous conscious planning. Whenever I hear myself say, "I am going to tell you a story," it is the signal for me to flip on my tape recorder.

Last of all, I am convinced that effective therapy through storytelling depends on the therapist's willingness to trust his or her own creativity and intuition, his willingness to open himself up to his own unconscious and to allow it to take over. When we can trust our unconscious, then our creativity flowers and proliferates. The books and tapes about Milton Erickson's anecdotes are a metaphor for our own inventiveness. It is not enough to offer pallid imitations of his stories; rather, we need to use his teachings as a springboard to catapult us into our own creativity. I hope that these stories will encourage others to tell their own stories in their own way to the "third ear."

Author's note to those who may imagine that they recognize themselves or others in the following case histories and stories: The names and sometimes the gender of the clients in the following case histories which accompany the stories have been changed to preserve professional confidentiality. In some instances I have told the stories to more than one client when the metaphor suited their case histories, and so, the "client" who is described sometimes is not a single person but a composite of two or more people.

Because I find it awkward to write he/she, I have chosen to arbitrarily assign gender throughout. In any story, gender can be changed at will, of course, and I do so freely whenever it is appropriate.

1

Porky the Porcupine

(A Story for a
Paranoid Personality)

Arnold sat as far from me as he could without actually rearranging the furniture. He spoke in a subdued monotone, with his gaze fixed on the carpet between his feet. He mumbled the name of one of my clients, saying she had suggested that he come to see me. After some hesitation, he said that she was the reason he decided to come. He told me that he was in love with her, but she had another boyfriend, and had no time for him except as a "friend." He had been spending most of his time fantasizing about her, and he was feeling "upset and nervous all the time."

Slowly his tale of loneliness unfolded. He was 21 years old. He worked as a belt-line assembler in a factory at night. He preferred night jobs because "people don't bother me then." He dropped out of college his freshman year, although he had been a straight A student in high school, because he got in with a "bad bunch" and spaced out on beer and marijuana. No "chick" had ever looked at him twice. He still lived at home with his parents and three brothers. He had "fixed up" the basement so no one would bother him, and he could "space out" whenever he pleased. He spent a great deal of time having sexual fantasies about women. Right now they were about Sylvia, the one who referred him to me. He thought that maybe I could help him with Sylvia.

His appearance was bizarre. His long blonde hair was unwashed, tied back in a ponytail with a rubber band; his teeth were prominent with pointed bicuspids, longer than his front teeth, lending him an animal-like appearance of ferocity; he also was at least 50 pounds overweight.

In ensuing sessions Arnold talked about feeling ugly. Frequently his fantasies centered around a "Beauty and the Beast" theme. He was convinced that his coworkers whispered about him, and when they laughed together he "knew" they were talking and laughing about him. He felt suspicious of everyone, was constantly alert to possible insult, and was ready for a fight on the slightest real or imagined provocation. Most of all, he was afraid.

Arnold resisted going into trance for several months. But gradually he learned to trust me. I saw him individually on the average of once a week, mainly working toward rapport and trust. He finally agreed to join one of the groups which met with me weekly, although he was reluctant to risk it. In the group there were both men and women about his own age. He lost no time obsessively fixing his attention on one of the young women there. When she would not respond to his phone calls, or his unscheduled appearances at her door, he began acting out in group. He sulked, he glared angrily at her, he muttered under his breath, and sometimes he skipped sessions. But as the weeks passed, he observed the work of others in the group (which he decided was all prearranged by me in order for him to understand his problems). He began to make a few changes. He got a haircut. He began to clean himself up. But he continued to fix his gaze on the carpet between his feet, and he spoke only when directly addressed.

When at last we succeeded in inducing trance, he began to relax somewhat. And after almost a year of work, the following story told itself.

O nce upon a time, there was a little porcupine. He was a very strange looking creature because although he had quite a small body, it was covered from head to foot with many long fierce-looking quills, and they stuck up all around his body, even when they were lying down, so the little porcupine looked three times his real size. And that was very useful to him because when he would go walking out of his burrow where he lived, he noticed that other animals and birds, much larger than he, would stop when they saw him and give him a wide berth. He thought that was very funny, but also he felt a little sad because he felt quite lonely, and he didn't know any other porcupines. And so he had to spend a lot of time alone. When he walked, he saw that other creatures seemed to be afraid of him and that seemed very strange to him, because HE was afraid of THEM. As a matter of fact, if there would be a sudden loud noise, or some creature would come up behind him suddenly, then, without trying at all, every quill on his body would stand straight up, and he would look not just three times his size, but ten times his size, and other creatures would back off. Sometimes they would say to him, "My goodness, you're fierce. My goodness, you're an angry one. Why are you so angry?" And the little porcupine was puzzled because he didn't feel angry at all. He just felt scared. And he did notice that from time to time when some foolish creature would get too close, his quills would stick in them, and they would run off screeching and hollering and crying when he had done nothing but stand still. Other creatures accused him of shooting his quills at them. It wasn't true at all. All he would do is stand still, and they would come up and get stuck, and then they would be angry and hurt because they said he had attacked them. All of this was very, very puzzling to the little porcupine. And so his days passed, and he felt very confused and very lonely and quite bored because he couldn't

22

think of anything for a little porcupine to do by himself that might be interesting.

One day as he was walking in the forest, as usual going his own lonely way, he met a huge turtle, and the turtle stopped and looked at him and said, "My goodness, you're a strange looking one." And Porky raised up all his quills at once because he felt very afraid. And the turtle said, "That is amazing! You can make yourself ten times your size whereas all I can do is pull my head and feet in and make myself smaller." "Oh," said the porcupine. "let me see!" And so the turtle obligingly pulled his head in and pulled in his feet, and, in fact, he was much smaller, and not only that, he looked so much like the rocks and stones all about him that the porcupine had to look very closely to see which one was the turtle. "My," said the porcupine, "I wish I could pull in my head and feet and make myself into a stone." And the turtle peeked out and said, "Oh, I wish I could make myself ten times as big, and have those fierce-looking spears all over me, instead of having to pull in and be like a stone. It's dark in there and very boring." "Well," said the porcupine, "you know something, I'm bored too because with my making myself ten times as big as I am and sticking out my fierce-looking quills, all other creatures avoid me." "Well," said the turtle, "that's very strange. I wouldn't want to avoid you. Why do they avoid you?" "Well," said the porcupine, "if they come near, they get hurt." "Ha, ha, ha," said the turtle. "I can come near." And he did. And the little porcupine began to shake because no other creature had ever come so close. And the turtle said, "See, I can even touch you." And he did. And the porcupine backed off and said, "Ooh, don't touch me! Nobody has ever touched me!" But the turtle said, "I can touch you." And the porcupine said, "So you can. And my quills don't stick into you." "Oh, no," said the turtle, "because I have this beautiful shell. See my beautiful shell? Oh, yes . . . yes," said the turtle, "you have your quills and I have my shell, and those protect us because inside we're really soft and very scared." And the little porcupine began to laugh because he had found a friend who understood exactly how he felt and was not afraid of his quills, and he was not afraid of the turtle because the turtle was not afraid of him. And do you know, they became very good friends.

Then the little porcupine began to understand that everyone else was afraid like him, and so he learned to keep his quills sleek against his body even though his heart was beating very hard. And ever after when he would meet a new creature, he kept his fierce-looking quills sleek against his body so he looked only three times his real size instead of ten times. And he learned to say, "Are you afraid? Because I'm afraid too, but all I want to do is play. Is that what you want?" And do you know, the next time he met a little chipmunk, the chipmunk said, "Yes, that's how I feel too, and do you mean that you won't shoot your spears at me if I come close?" "Of course not," said the porcupine, "and anyway, I can't shoot any spears. I can only make them stand up and you get stuck if you come too close when I'm afraid." "Oh," said the chipmunk, "you don't have to be afraid of me. All I can do is scratch and bite and there is no place on you at all where I could bite or scratch. You don't have to be afraid of me, and if you won't stick me with your quills, I don't have to be afraid of you." "That's right," said the porcupine, and laughed out loud with pleasure, and do you know, soon the little porcupine was friends with everyone in the forest.

One day, a surly big creature came into the forest. No one had ever seen anyone like him before. When he laughed it sounded like a snarl, and when he snarled he sounded even worse, and he was very ugly, although no one wanted him to know that they thought so. He had long front legs and sort of crouching, cringing back legs, and he had ugly rough fur in patches, and a long mean snoot, and long snaggly teeth. This creature came swaggering up to where the little porcupine was standing with all his quills sleek against his body. The little porcupine said, "Hello," in a quavering voice. The creature laughed his laugh which sounded like a snarl, and the little porcupine asked, "What is your name?" The creature said, "What's it to ya?" "Oh," said the little porcupine, "my name is Porky." And the creature laughed like a snarl again. "And I would like to know your name," said Porky. "Oh, well, all right, nosey," he said. "My name is Laughing Hyena." "Oh," said Porky, "that's an interesting name." "You making fun of me?" snarled the hyena, and Porky cried, "Oh, no sir, no sir. Not at all, sir." "Well," said the laughing hyena, "you'd better not because I could just make mincemeat outa you in one bite." Little Porky's quills stood straight up, and the laughing hyena said, "Oh, you wanta fight, do ya? Well, I'll show you." And so he jumped at little Porky, and little Porky stood there shaking and shaking all over like a thistle in the wind. And do you know what happened? That mean laughing hyena got his long mean snoot stuck full of quills and there were quills sticking in his ears and all over his ugly body. He put his tail between his legs and ran off howling hideously, straight out of the forest. Then all the creatures applauded and said, "Oh, Porky, you were wonderful." And Porky said, "Well, I really didn't do anything. And I feel bad now because I did what I just have learned not to do. I have learned not to scare off everyone, and to realize that everyone is scared of me." "That's all right, Porky," they said, "there are times when you have to use what you have to protect yourself but most of the time you just have to be friends." And little Porky felt glad in his heart because from then on he knew the difference between making friends and protecting himself.

The story marked a definite turning point for Arnold. Shortly after that session, he enrolled in a computer programming course of study at the university. He joined a ballroom dancing class there. Eventually he met a young woman who became his lover. He went regularly to a gymnasium for weightlifting exercises. He learned to swim. Then he bought his first "dress up" clothes, a blazer and slacks. Next he arranged for a dentist to even his teeth. He began to like his appearance. He discovered that he possessed a wry sense of humor to which people responded. He changed to a daytime job, and eventually moved into a job designing software for computers.

Our sessions continued for about a year, in which we used trance to reinforce and further his changes. Now I see Arnold about twice a year. He is planning to get married in a few months.

2

The Green Dragon

(A Story for the
Treatment of Phobia)

Andrew arrived at my office exuding nervous energy. Well-dressed in a too-studied correlation of matching colors and textures, he wore a large diamond ring on the little finger of his right hand. In a rapid-fire burst of words he began defending himself for coming to consult with me. He explained that he felt silly about seeing a "shrink." It seemed that his difficulties were "absurd and quite uncomplicated," but often he felt uncomfortable and seemed to be getting worse.

Andrew was employed as the head designer for a large, well-known clothing factory which manufactured high-style, extremely expensive dresses. Not only did he have full responsibility for the "line," but his duties included personally presiding over all fashion presentations to buyers. This involved six major fashion showings a year in such centers as New York, as well as Texas, California, and the Midwest. This had always been difficult for him, but lately he was experiencing more and more difficulty in standing up and speaking before an audience, so much so that he had begun faking sickness as an excuse for failing to appear. His boss was becoming impatient with him. He was afraid he might lose his job in disgrace. Yes, he had tried various means to deal with his panic, ranging the gamut from stimulants to "downers," but nothing seemed to work.

In the weeks that followed, he unfolded his story—a tale of insecurity and a deep sense of inadequacy. He often felt like an imposter and was afraid he would be exposed as a fake, be ridiculed and laughed out of his field. Although he tried harder and harder for perfection, he was filled with self-hatred because he seemed never to achieve it. About this time, among the many details Andrew related to me, he mentioned from time to time that he was disturbed by a recurring dream about a green dragon.

Andrew's resistance to hypnosis was persistent. It took more than two months for him to be able to relax and begin to trust me. His frequent protest was, "I feel so ridiculous." But gradually he was able to let go of his fear sufficiently to go into a light trance. I taught him to hypnotize himself, which worked better for him. He was making noticeable progress when the following story told itself.

O nce upon a time there was a little boy who was very, very rich. He was so rich that he had a special room, a large room just for his toys and treasures. And he would go there every day. Now you would think that he would be a very, very happy little boy, with so very many toys and treasures, but that was not the case. Actually, the little boy was very, very sad because although he had many beautiful toys and many, many treasures, there was one thing that spoiled everything for him. Sitting over in the corner of the room, barely visible behind all the heaped-up toys and treasures, sat a large, green dragon. And this dragon never seemed to take its eyes off the little boy. And no matter what the little boy was doing, whenever he looked up, there he would see the green dragon watching him. And this would spoil his fun because in his heart, he was very, very afraid of the dragon. He would dream that the green dragon would rush upon him, throw him down, and try to kill him. And every night the little boy would wake up screaming. He never would or could explain to anyone about his nightmare because he was afraid that the green dragon would get him if he told. And so he felt very, very unhappy. He was so unhappy that sometimes he would dance and play very hard, and whirl around and laugh very loudly, and talk a blue streak, thinking that would make him forget about the dragon in the corner. But do you know that no matter how loudly he laughed, how hard he played or how fast he danced and whirled and jumped, when he stopped, he would look in the corner and there would be the green dragon still staring at him, still looking very, very menacing. The little boy would sit down feeling dejected and quiet. His fun would be spoiled again. And this state of affairs went on for a very long time. Each day, the little boy would begin the day playing with his toys, happily trying to forget about the green dragon, and each day he would end the day sitting quiet and sad with the tears running down his face.

One day, a friend came to visit the boy. The visitor was another boy his very same age and size. The new boy looked around the room with eyes opening wider and wider and said, "Oh, what wonderful treasures." And he ran around picking up this one and that one and playing and clapping his hands, but the little rich boy felt anxious and worried. He kept stealing glances at the green dragon. He did not join his friend. Suddenly, to his horror, he saw his friend run over to the dragon and start to sit astride him. The little boy cried, "NO, NO, don't do that." And his friend said, "Why ever not?" "Oh," said the little boy, "he is such a fierce and ugly dragon. Surely he will harm you because I know he tries to harm me. I am so afraid of him." "Ho, ho, ho," said his little friend, "look at

30

this." And he turned the dragon so the little boy could see, and there down the back of the dragon was a long, shiny zipper. The little boy didn't know what to make of that. He watched with round eyes, still trembling with fear. And his friend said, "You want to see?" But the little boy said, "I'm not sure, I'm not sure." So his friend said, "Nonsense," and unzipped the dragon. And do you know, the whole dragon's green suit fell down. And what do you think was in there? Another little boy! This little boy laughed, stood up and said, "Oh, ho, ho, I enjoyed being a dragon until I was discovered. All this time I had such fun spooking and making you afraid."

And the little boy said, "That was very mean of you. Why did you do it?" "Oh," said the ex-dragon, I did it because it was such fun. You had so many treasures, so many things, if you hadn't had any dragons among them, how would you have known how lucky you are?" "Oh," the little boy said, and stamped his foot, "that's nonsense. That's nonsense. That was mean of you to pretend to be a dragon all the time and zip yourself up in that dragon suit, and here you are, just another little boy like me."

Then the three friends began laughing together and said to each other, "It was fun." Then can you guess what they did? They took turns zipping themselves up in the dragon suit and scaring each other. They pretended to be, ooooh, very afraid of the dragon, and then they pretended to kill the dragon, and then the dragon pretended to kill them, and all the time they were laughing and having such sport.

At last the little boy clapped his hands and said, "Now we can have fun with all my treasures." And so they did, but the best fun was playing dragon, and that remained one of their favorite games. Now the little boy was happy. He played with all his treasures and shared them with his friends, and he loved having his new friends. Soon word spread in the countryside about his marvelous treasures. More little girls and boys came because they heard of the wonderful toys, but best of all they heard about the dragon suit. They came to pretend with the dragon and to play the dragon game. Some children asked, "Where can I find a dragon suit for myself?" and they were told, "Why, you can make one up yourself." And the little boy said, "I think I understand because I think I did make one up myself. What I didn't know was that it has a zipper and the dragon suit can come off."

After the story, Andrew could allow himself to go into trance easily and deeply. In the following three months he focused on visualizing his considerable talent as a designer. He rehearsed his speeches in trance, visualized his success at forthcoming presentations, and augmented his creativity by calling on his "creative unconscious" for ideas. He learned to relax into his anxiety and use it to energize his performance.

When last I heard, Andrew was actually enjoying his public appearances.

3

The Little Clock That Couldn't Tell Time

(A Story for a Schizophrenic
With Obsessive-compulsive Disorder)

*W*hen Martha came into my office she sat nervously rubbing her hands as though washing them. Her unusually light blue eyes seemed curiously vacant, and her face lacked expression. She wore a faded print scarf tied over her head, completely hiding her hair. Her clothes were several sizes too large, lending her an appearance of flat-chested frailty. She wore men's shoes, shabby and much too big for her. Her large-knuckled hands were red and swollen like those of a dishwasher.

Martha had difficulty telling me about herself. It required many sessions for her to relate bits and pieces of her difficulties. She was 26 years old. She lived alone in a single room in a poor neighborhood. She liked to save things like newspapers, and even though the small room was very crowded, she could not bring herself to throw anything away. Her mother visited her weekly, taking the dirty laundry home and bringing fresh bedsheets and clothes. Mother insisted on cleaning the room which upset Martha who, nevertheless, could not confront her parent. And as she worked, mother scolded her daughter during the entire visit. Martha dreaded the visits. Even more, she dreaded the times she was required to visit her mother and older sister, who shared a house. She felt ashamed there because they criticized her for spending so much time in the bathroom washing her hands. Later I learned that she washed her hands almost continuously. But only her hands, because she was afraid to get into the bathtub.

Her eating and sleeping habits were erratic. She ate very

little, with no planning about provisions. Sometimes she subsisted on tea alone for days. There were no set meal times. She stayed awake for most of the night, unwilling to lie down. Martha complained that her feet were swollen and painful from standing on them for long periods. She spent her nights playing her guitar and "making up" songs. She had no friends but she talked to people on the street sometimes and on the bus coming to my office. She wondered about joining the Hare Krishna religion.

She maintained herself on disability insurance. She had never been able to hold a job because she felt incapable of arriving anywhere on time. Sometimes she would arrive at my office as much as 45 minutes late for her appointment. At such times I would see her for five minutes. Sometimes she didn't make it at all, and at other times she would come 45 minutes early.

After more than a month had passed, Martha told me the reason she was coming to see me. Her mother had threatened to put her into the state hospital unless she went for treatment. Martha agreed to come to see me in the hope that I would prevent her mother from committing her. I suggested that she ask her mother to join our sessions. Martha was reluctant, but after a few weeks finally agreed to my telephoning her mother. She proved to be most willing to come in. A stout, gray-haired woman with a blunt way of speaking and a righteous manner, she had difficulty in hiding her hostility. In Martha's presence she expressed her anger toward her daughter for "not trying," for dirty habits and slovenly ways. She complained that Martha would "live in filth like an animal" if mother did not come to clean up each week. I suggested that it was loving of her to want to help Martha, and it certainly helped Martha stay in touch with her mother. Underneath it all, I said, I could tell they both cared very much about each *other. And perhaps they could think of some new ways that might work better to show their wish to stay connected. Martha watched me big-eyed and confused. Mother hesitated but remained unconvinced. She telephoned just before their next appointment to say that she could see no improvement in Martha whatsoever and was not willing to come in with her anymore.*

It was true that Martha did not show any signs of change. But she did continue to come. I began to use hypnotherapy and stories in treating her. She liked to experience trance, and she enjoyed the stories. But there were no noticeable results . . . until I told the following story.

O nce upon a time there was a pretty little clock that lived in a pretty little room in a very pretty little house. The little clock would tick merrily on, and its shining face was so bright that it actually sounded happy and looked happy where it lived on the top of the bureau. And there it went tick tock tick tock tick tock, singing a little song, all day and all night. Now in this pretty little house there was a housekeeper, and she had a very heavy step so that when she walked the whole room would shake a little. Her movements were very brisk, very vigorous, and most often she had a little frown on her face. Her lips were pursed because she had so many things to do that she felt very, very hurried. Perhaps she was even a little angry that she had so much to do. But in any case, she was very, very much in a hurry, and she would come into the center of the room, put her hands on her hips and look around, pursing her lips and frowning. Then she would walk heavily over to the bureau, pick up the little clock and wind it, hard. Wind grind, wind grind, wind grind, and then set it down sharply on top of the bureau again. The little clock would lose a tick or two but then would settle down again and soon forget the shaking up when the housekeeper left the room.

But one day, the housekeeper came in and seemed in even more of a hurry than ever. And this time, she wound the little clock too tight. And the little clock stopped ticking. It simply sat there silent and sad. The next day, the housekeeper came into the room again with a bang and a burst, strode over to the bureau, looked at the little clock and said, "Tsk, tsk. Tsk, tsk. This no-good little clock has stopped ticking." And so she shook it, and shook it again, listened, put it to her ear, stood back and peered at it, set it down again smartly, and shaking her head and frowning with disapproval, walked out of the room again. The next day she came in and did the same thing, and on the third day, she picked up the little clock, walked heavily over to the closet, stuck it on the top shelf, dusted off her hands and said, "Well, that's that," and shut the closet door. There the little clock sat silent and unhappy for what seemed like a very long time, when one day, the closet door opened, and the housekeeper stood there looking over all the contents of the closet, spied the little clock on the top shelf, and exclaimed, "Well, I forgot about that." She lifted the clock down, looked at it, shook it again and then, frowning, she said, "This clock is of no more use," and tossed the little clock in the wastebasket. The little clock had a heavy heart indeed, a very heavy heart. Also, it was afraid. Later that day, the wastebasket was carried out of the house and dumped into the trash bin and there the little clock lay, exposed to the air and the rain and the sun until the trash collector came later that week. And he collected the trash. The little clock lay there in the middle of all the discarded junk, and when he got to the dump, he threw the little clock and all the other bits and pieces, odds and ends, into the dump. And the little clock thought, "Oooh, this is the end of me." And so silently it lay there in the trash.

One bright morning, it seemed especially bright because it was spring, the little clock heard light footsteps and heard a cheerful, small voice saying, "What a pretty little clock. Whatever is it doing here?" And the little clock felt itself being lifted up and gently held. Suddenly hope sprang, a little gleam of hope sprang inside. It was a little girl holding the pretty clock, and she turned it this way and that, upside down and all around. She shook it a little, gently. She tried to wind it carefully, but she saw that the little clock could not tell time. Yet it was so pretty that she decided to take it home with her anyway, and when she got it home, she put it on the little bedside table beside her bed, and sat there looking at the face of the pretty little clock, wondering what she might do so the little clock could tell time again. And then she remembered that down the street, there was a clockmaker's shop, and in the shop there was an old clockmaker. "Oh," she said, "perhaps he can fix my pretty little clock." And so without waiting another second, she picked it up and ran as fast as she could down the block to the clockmaker's shop. She walked in and looked about, and it was a sight and a sound to behold. There seemed to be hundreds of clocks all over the walls, all ticking in a different time, all chiming in a different tune, and there was such a symphony, such an orchestra of ticking and tocking and chiming and ringing that she had to laugh out loud with delight. At the far end of the shop, with his back to her, sat a very old man. And as she approached him slowly, wondering what to say, he turned suddenly and said in a deep voice, "Well, what have we got here?" And the little girl held out her pretty little clock and said, "Please, sir, this pretty little clock doesn't tell time anymore. It can't keep time anymore. Could you possibly fix it?" "Well," said the old clockmaker, "let me see." And he looked at it and he turned it around and he lifted off its little back cover and peered in. "Well, well, well," he said, "someone has wound this little clock too tightly." And then he peered at the little girl over his spectacles and said, "I will see what I can do, but I cannot promise you anything. Sometimes a little clock can be fixed, and sometimes not. So you come back in three days, and then I will let you know." "Oh, thank you, sir, thank you, sir," said the little girl. "That is so kind of you. Thank you." And she turned and ran out the door, but when she got outside, she stopped and slowly turned to look back into the shop, and her heart was beating very hard as she began thinking anxiously, "Oh, I do hope he can fix my pretty little clock. Oh, I do hope he can fix my pretty little clock so it can tell time again." And she walked slowly home, dragging one foot and then the other, now and then walking a little more quickly, and now and then stopping and thinking very hard. When she got in, she said, "Oh, if only the clockmaker can fix my little clock, I will be ever so good from now on. I will make my bed every morning carefully, without being told or scolded. I will brush my teeth in the morning and at bedtime without being told or asked. I will pick up my clothes from the floor and hang them away neatly. I will go to bed on time and my little clock will tell me. I will do everything I know I ought to do. I will be a very, very good girl. I will keep my room ever so neat, and I will be on time for everything if only I have my little clock to tell me when."

The three days passed very slowly, very slowly. They seemed like three weeks. Sometimes the hours seemed like three hours. Sometimes the days semed like three days, each one. But at last, they passed, and when it was time, the little girl hurried down to the clockmaker's shop and opened the door.

Suddenly, she felt afraid to go in. She felt afraid to hear what the clockmaker would tell her. But, at last, she took a deep breath and walked in, standing straight and trying to look brave. She walked straight up to the clockmaker, who had his back turned to her again, and she stood there, but he didn't turn around. Finally, she coughed a little and said, "Excuse me, sir." The clockmaker raised his head and said, "What? What's that?" He said, "Who? What, what's that?" She said, "Excuse me, sir." And he turned and peered at her over his shoulder. "What is it, little girl? What is it?" And she said, "Well, excuse me, sir, but have you fixed my little clock?" And he said, "Little clock? Fixed your little clock? What little clock?" Oh, and her heart sank. Oh, what if her little clock was lost? What if he had forgotten? What if he couldn't fix it after all? And so she said, "You remember, sir, three days ago, I brought a pretty little clock, and you said it was wound too tight? And you would see if you could fix it and to come back in three days? Well, it has been three days." "Oh, sure enough, sure enough, let me see." And he got up, slowly, and walked stiffly to a little cupboard, opened the cupboard, reached in, and brought out the pretty little clock. "Well," he said, "is this the one?" And the little girl jumped up and down and said, "Yes, sir, yes, sir. that's the one." He said, "Well, then, here it is ticking away, merrily ticking away." "Oooh, sir," said the little girl, "thank you, thank you, sir." And she looked into the clock's face and the little clock seemed to smile back at her, and its pretty hands were pointing exactly to the right time, and its little tick was steady, soft, and musical. The little girl hugged the clock to her, looked up into the old clockmaker's eyes, and said, "Thank you for fixing my little clock." And so she ran home, and put her merry little clock that could now tell time again, she put it on her bedside table, and there they lived together happily ever after.

After the story, Martha became noticeably more relaxed and trusting. She began to follow suggestions about eating and resting. Eventually she enrolled in a city-supported rehabilitation program to acquire some job skills. She enjoyed the group sessions at the rehab center and even began to feel a sense of belonging there. She began to clean herself up. She accepted a part-time job doing simple yardwork that I had arranged for her. I told stories about the earth being "clean" dirt, and how putting her hands in it was healthy and good. She began to make an attempt to arrive on time. There were numerous backslidings, but on the whole she was making good changes.

One day, after more than a year had passed, Martha asked me about a famous nearby clinic for residential care. She had heard that it was a place very different from the state hospital, a place where people like her got better. We talked about it. For a long time I had been thinking about suggesting residential care for Martha, but up until then had not been able to allay her terror of institutions. I asked if she thought she might like to go there to live for a while. To my surprise she asked me to discuss it with her mother. Her mother was pleased that her daughter would consider going to an institution. She knew how terrified Martha had been by the very idea. And in time, arrangements were made for her to go. Martha has been in treatment there for more than a year.

4

The Little Centipede Who Didn't Know How to Walk

(A Story for an Obsessive-compulsive
Personality Disorder)

*P*eter arrived 20 minutes early for his appointment. When I asked him to come into my office, he looked at his watch, gathered up his books and his coat, but seemed hesitant to accept my invitation. Finally, he got up, looked back at the waiting room exit, looked at me, responded to my encouraging nod with a sick smile, and followed me into my office. There he sat passively looking at the backs of his hands.

His story unfolded slowly and painfully. Orphaned by an automobile accident when he was still an infant, he was reared by a maiden aunt, his mother's older sister. It seems she was an exemplary person who adhered strictly to her Christian code of ethics. And she firmly parented Peter to do the same. He "owed a great deal to her." He had been a good student in school, but he seemed to need much more time to complete his work than did the others. He thought it was because he carefully organized everything before he started to study, and carefully checked his work several times before turning it in. His standards always had been very high and he believed that "whatever is worth doing is worth doing well." His aunt seemed to expect excellence from him, and took it for granted that he would bring home "A's." And if on occasion he reported a lesser grade, for example a "90" on an arithmetic assignment, she would ask, "What happened to the other ten?" His ambition had always been to get an "A" in everything he undertakes. No, he didn't have much time for friends. Actually, he had found most of his peers to be silly and frivolous. They wasted a lot of time fooling around, and were shockingly care-less about how they used their money. His aunt had taught him to save his money in an orderly fashion.

Last year (his twenty-first), his aunt died of a heart attack. He felt bewildered and lost. Although he worked harder and longer at his job as a bookkeeper, and although he enrolled in night classes at the university, still he felt anxious and unhappy. One night he met a young lady named Mary Ann at the university. Mary Ann was his aunt's name also. They had been spending every Wednesday evening and Saturday afternoon together for more than nine months. Mary Ann wanted to get married. But Peter thought they needed to get to know each other much better before making such an im-portant decision. He thought that they should continue as they were for at least two years in order to be sure they were "right" for each other. Mary Ann felt angry about it. And now when he had to work overtime on Wednesdays or Saturdays and was late for their meetings, Mary Ann was beginning to behave unpleasantly.

He had been thinking about coming in to consult with me for at least three months, but could not make up his mind whether or not that would be the right thing to do. When Mary Ann told him last week that she had decided not to con-tinue their meetings, he felt very upset and decided to arrange an appointment with me. He started to cancel the appoint-ment yesterday, but then changed his mind. Actually, he had changed his mind back and forth several times. Did I think I could help him? We made another appointment. As he put his hand on the doorknob to leave, he said, "By the way, I forgot to tell you that for about six months I find myself count-ing in my head, over and over. First I count to one hundred, and then I count from one hundred backwards to one again. I seem to be doing it more and more with each passing day."

In the months that followed, Peter began to respond slowly to positive reinforcement and empathy. He liked the ritual of listening to the relaxation tape we made. His episodes of compulsive counting grew less frequent. Mary Ann agreed to meet with him again although not on a regular basis. He discovered that his episodes of counting occurred when Mary Ann became "aggressive" and tried to kiss or hug.

We began hypnotherapy. It was slow work at first. Even when it was clearly apparent to me that Peter was in trance, he continued to protest that actually he was not in trance but had merely fallen asleep, and that the therapy was not working. But gradually he stopped his counting and finally even decided to plan a day-long bicycle trip with Mary Ann and her friends away from his books and his job. At this point the following story appeared.

O nce upon a time, there was a little centipede who got separated from his parents. And he was separated when he was so young that the poor little centipede had not yet had time to learn to walk. He was in a terrible, terrible predicament trying to teach all of his hundred legs to work together so that he could walk. And he had been trying for a very long time but somehow when his front legs would go in one direction, his middle ones would go in another, and his hind legs would go yet in a third, fourth and sometimes even in a sixth direction, until finally he would just crumble into a little ball of despair wondering how on earth he was ever going to get to bed because he was so tired and his bed was all the way across the room — a long room that, measured in centipede size, looked like a hundred miles long. And so for the hundredth time, he stood up and looked down at his two rows of feet and said, "Now, feet, you listen to me! First, the right side will move forward and STOP, and then the left side will move forward and STOP." And both sides said, "No, that's not how it goes. It's 'Right and Wrong,' 'Right and Wrong.' And you say, 'Right and left,' and that isn't it. I don't want to be left. And I don't want to be wrong. I want to be right." And the centipede said, "OH, NO, NOT AGAIN. I've explained that to you a HUNDRED TIMES." It seems that everything that the little centipede did was measured by the number of feet he had. "So, now, for the hundredth time, I want the LEFT side . . . " "No," said the left side, "that's the wrong side." "Oh!" said the centipede in exasperation. "All right, then, RIGHT SIDE, FORWARD MARCH, and STOP." So one side went forward and then he said, "Now, left side . . . " "NO," they said. "When will you learn? It's not that. It's 'Right and Wrong.' Everybody knows it's 'Right and Wrong.' And we're not wrong. We're RIGHT. So you just call us 'RIGHT' and then we'll move." "Oh," said the centipede, "this is impossible. How am I ever going to learn to walk when these stupid feet keep mixing me up with RIGHT AND LEFT and RIGHT AND WRONG until I don't know myself WHAT IS RIGHT FROM WRONG." "Oh," he said, "even I am doing it now."

And while he was sitting down, with all hundred feet splayed out around him like a fringe, he heard a voice from above him. He looked up and there he saw a big old wise spider. And the spider said, "What's the trouble, little fellow?" And the centipede explained that his stupid feet wanted to fight about right and wrong, and would not move right and left feet in turn, and that no amount of explaining would get it through their stupid feet . . . heads . . . feet . . . feet . . . yes, that's right, feet.

And the spider began to laugh, and he said, "You know, I understand. I have only six feet, but I remember that when I was little, it was very hard for me to sort out which foot ought to go first, and which foot ought to go next, and what was the order in which they needed to go." "Oh," said the centipede, "perhaps that will help." So he said, "Okay, everybody, stand up." And so they all stood up. "Now," he said, "right proceed forward, left . . . " "Oh, no," said the left. "Wrong." He said, "No, left." They said, "No, wrong. What's right is that we want to be right. We don't want to be left. We can't be left behind. It would be stupid for you to just go forward. You would JUST TURN AROUND IN A CIRCLE. Did you ever think of that?"

And the centipede looked in despair at the spider, and the spider was laughing and shaking his sides. "Oh, I see what the trouble is. They have mixed up HOW TO GO with what is RIGHT AND WRONG, and IT HAS NOTHING TO DO WITH RIGHT OR WRONG. It has only to do with going first one side then the other, one side then the other, and then they make a team. And then they go in the same direction, all together, and join in the same effort. And when they understand that, then they'll be ABLE TO PROCEED." So the little centipede said, "But how can I ever make them understand that? You know they absolutely insist that it's what it should be or it shouldn't be, and that right and wrong is what is at issue, and I explained that it's right and left . . . " "NO, no," said the left side, "no, no, we don't want to get left, that's the whole point. You have misunderstood us again. We are not going to get left. We want to go right with all the others. Right on, with them." "Oh," the centipede groaned, "you hear?"

And the spider said, "Well, look, let me show you." And so he got up in front, and he looked over his spider shoulder, and he said to the centipede, "Okay, now you over here," and he pointed with one of his right legs, "move forward, one, two, three, stop. RIGHT?" The others said, "RIGHT!" And he looked on the other side, and he said, "Now, you over here," and he pointed to the left, "you move forward, one, two, three, right?" They said, "Yes! Now that's it." He said, "So, good. You're both right. Right, right. Right, right. Forward march. Right, right. GOOD. No one gets left. Everyone's right. Good." And before he knew it, the little centipede had reached his bed, and he turned, and he said, "Thank you very much, sir. That was very helpful, and I'll remember that all I need to remember is that all my feet are RIGHT, then NO ONE can be WRONG, and everyone will do what's RIGHT." And the spider looked at him and winked and said, "Right!"

After the story Peter continued in therapy for about another year. Gradually he learned to balance his time better between work and play. He allowed himself to laugh from time to time. He took a vacation when his classes ended. He began to feel sexually attracted to Mary Ann. When we terminated treatment he wanted to know if I thought that long engagements were the wisest, or did I think it is okay for people to be married very soon.

5

Twins

(A Story for a Passive-Aggressive
Personality Disorder)

*W*hen Trudy telephoned for an appointment, she wanted to discuss whether or not I thought she needed therapy. No, she had never seen a therapist before, although she had telephoned several therapists from time to time, but always had changed her mind, and put it off. She said that one time she did go for one appointment, but decided the therapist didn't like her so she never went back. After some pulling and hauling, she made an appointment with me. But she did not show up, and she did not call to cancel. Almost a week later she telephoned with a story about running out of gas on her way to my office. By the time she got help (it seems that passersby deliberately ignored her), it was too late to come. Then she failed to telephone because she was afraid I would be angry. She hoped I would give her a second chance – if not, well, then . . . . Her tone implied a defiant "so what?"

On the day of her appointment she arrived 20 minutes late. She appeared to be in her mid-thirties with a rather heavy face, prominent nose, and a permanent crease between her eyebrows. She was casually dressed in shabby jeans and a loose sweater. Immediately she launched into blaming her boss for her tardiness. She described him as unreasonably demanding and unappreciative. No matter what she did to try to please him, it was never good enough. And if sometimes she did make a mistake – after all she is only human – he would throw a fit. Yes, since she was a skilled typist she had little trouble finding work.

She described her relationship with her lover of three years' standing, a description which bore striking similarities to her complaints about her boss. It seems that he expected her to be perfect. They quarreled often, and once he had hit her so hard that he broke her nose — all of this despite her constant efforts to please him. He got angry at the drop of a hat. Their apartment was never clean enough to suit him; her cooking wasn't good enough; heaven forbid if she sometimes should burn something a little, or if she sometimes forgot something; and heaven help her if she couldn't make up her mind instantly about a restaurant. Just like everyone else, sometimes she accidentally broke something or even misplaced something. He would fly into a rage. No wonder she would finally get fed up and refuse to sleep with him.

Her problem, she thought, was whether to stay with him or leave. She just could not make up her mind, so she just kept putting it off and putting it off. She doubted that coming for treatment would do much good. What did I think?

In our first few sessions we explored her past history. Child of divorced parents, she had been psychologically and physically abused by her alcoholic stepfather. Her mother was too frightened to protect her. Hungry for security and love, she learned to hide her feelings, especially her anger. Never had she dared to express her anger directly.

She was stuck in an endless repetitive litany of complaints and excuses. She skipped appointments. She arrived late. She had to be reminded to pay for her sessions. We began using trance early in her treatment, and after only six sessions, principally centered on nurturing and safety, the following story appeared.

O nce upon a time, there were two sisters, and they were twins. And though they looked exactly alike, they behaved in very different ways. One of them spent all her time thinking of ways to make people like her. She would rush to do things for people. She would try to help them. She would think of things to say that they would like. She would stop herself from saying what she thought they wouldn't like. She really was trying harder and harder to be very pleasing. Her twin was just the opposite. Her twin would say to people in an angry voice, "Why should I please you? YOU please ME! That's your job. Your job is to love me and make me feel good. I am not going to try to please you." She would do all kinds of angry things, just to see if she could make people prove that they were not going to be nice to her or love her for herself. And so these two had very different ways. The one who wanted everyone to love her often felt very hurt because the people would say, "Stop helping me! I can do this for myself. I don't want you to do this. Stop it." And she would feel very, very downcast and very hurt and think, "I was only trying to help you," and she was puzzled because she didn't get loved for always being so helpful. The other twin sometimes would meet someone who would laugh and say, "Oh, I'm not afraid of your temper and your angry words. What you need is a hug, and some loving." And to her surprise and puzzlement, she would get hugs instead of slaps and angry words. So both little girls often ended up very puzzled, not understanding at all how to behave.

One day as they were walking down the street, there in front of them they saw a charming little house. And the first sister said, "Would you like to go to the house over there and see who lives there?" And the other twin said, "You're always asking what I'd like to do. Well, what would you like to do? You decide for a change." And the other twin said, "Well, I was only trying to please you. I will do anything you want." And the other twin said, "Damn it, I'm sick of you saying you'll do anything I want. You decide once in a while what you want, and then I'll tell you if I'll do it or not." And so they kept on, back and forth, back and forth like that for at least five minutes, when they chanced to look up and saw standing there at the gate of the house a little old lady who was watching and listening. When she saw that she was noticed she said, "Little girls . . . ," and the little twin who liked to please said, "Yes, Ma'am?" And the little old lady said, "I couldn't help overhearing your quarrel, and I wondered if you would like to come inside and have a cup of tea with me." The first twin said, "Oh, that's very nice. May I help you fix it? I'll come in and I'll get the tea cups, and I'll make the tea, and I'll serve it." And the little old lady looked at her very seriously and said, "Please come in." Then the other twin said, "Well, I can imagine that I'm not going to like tea very much, but I'll give it a try and then I'll let you know."

And so they both went into the house with the little old lady. And the first twin said, "Where are the cups? Where is the kettle? What can I do to help?" The little old lady said, "I invited you for tea so please sit down. I will fix tea. I have done it many times. And I don't need help right now. If I should need help, I shall ask for it." The first little twin sat down and her heart sank as she thought, "Oh, I must have done something wrong again. But I was only trying to help. I don't know what I did wrong. Now that nice lady probably doesn't like me." And she felt like crying but she thought, "Oh, the little lady won't like it if I'm crying so I'll choke back my tears and not let her see." The other twin sat down and said, "Humph, the room's not bad, but there must be some trick here. Why does she want to give me tea? What has she got up her sleeve? And I'm not going to do what she wants. If she thinks she can con me into doing what she wants, she's got another think coming, but I won't let on. I'll just sit here and see."

Presently, the little old lady came back and she had a lovely shiny silver tray and on it were three of the prettiest little tea cups you can imagine. They were filled with fragrant tea, and she set the tray down as she said to the first little girl, "Do you take milk and sugar in your tea?" And the little girl said, "Oh, it doesn't matter. Anything you say." The old lady looked at her and said, "It's necessary for you to decide." And the little girl said, "I want to do what's right." Then the old lady said to her, "Ask yourself what you want. Trust yourself that it will be right."

And the little girl was afraid, but she asked herself, "What do I want?" And a little voice came up and said, "It's time you asked me. It's really time you asked me. What I want is sugar . . . two spoons. And some milk, if you please." The little girl said to the voice, "Hush, that's greedy! Two spoons! Are you sure one spoon's not enough? She might not like it." The little voice said, "She said for you to decide. I'm your decider." And the little girl said, "Oh," and she looked up at the old lady and she said, "I . . wo . . would . . like two spoons of sugar?" And she looked to see how the little old lady would react. The little old lady just smiled. "And some milk please . . . just a little." And the voice said, "I don't want 'just a little.' I want a lot." "Uh, oh, uh . . . a little more, please?" And the little old lady put a little more in and smiled at the little girl. And the little voice in the little girl said, "See," and the little girl took the cup of tea and waited for permission to drink it.

The little old lady turned to the other twin and said, "What would you like in your tea?" "Well," said the other one, "since you asked, it smells rather good the way it is, but maybe I'd better take some precautions. Please just put in one teaspoon of sugar. If I want more, I'll let you know." And the little old lady did as she was asked and handed the teacup to the little girl, who did not say thank you, just "hunh." And the little old lady put two teaspoons of sugar in her tea and filled it up with milk and they all sat down and began to sip their tea.

"Oh," said the first twin, "what a delicious cup of tea. Thank you, thank you so very much. Is it all right for me to drink it now?" And the little old lady looked straight in her eyes and said, "You don't need permission. What do YOU want to do?" And the little twin looked down and said to the voice inside her, "What do I want to do?" "Drink it, silly, drink it." So the little girl smiled at the old lady and said, "I have decided to drink it. Thank you." And the little old lady smiled at her and nodded. And the first twin thought, "Oh, she likes me when I decide myself, and she likes to decide herself, and she likes to do things for herself, and she likes to ask when she likes to ask, and not to ask when she doesn't like to ask. Oh, and I do like her, and you know, she smiled at me and I think she does like me."

The other little girl drank down her tea in one gulp to show that she didn't have to ask for anything, but she burned her tongue and her tongue felt awful, and she sputtered and she gasped and she said to the old lady, "The tea was too hot! Why did you give me such a hot cup of tea? I burned my tongue and it's your fault!" And the lady looked at her and said, "No, I didn't drink your tea and burn your tongue. You drank your tea and burned your tongue. So you decided to hurt yourself, not I." And the second twin sat and glowered and thought, "Everybody wants to say it's my fault. It's really their fault." And she sat and sulked. And she said, "I'm not going to ask that old lady for any more tea to burn my tongue. I have learned my lesson. That's what I get for trusting somebody. I knew I shouldn't have trusted her." So she sat and sulked.

Then the little old lady said to them, "I noticed that the two of you are very different. I noticed too that you wear the same shoes and that you look exactly alike. But I noticed that you . . . ," and she looked at the first twin, " . . . are wearing a pink dress, and I noticed that you . . . ," and she looked at the other twin, " . . . are wearing a blue dress." And she said to the first twin, "I noticed that you are wearing a blue jacket, and I noticed," as she looked at the other twin, "that you are wearing a pink jacket. Now I'm wondering if you'd be willing to trade jackets." And the first twin looked at the little old lady and said sweetly, "Is that what you want me to do?" And the second twin glowered at her and said gruffly, "Why should I do that? I don't want her old jacket. I like my jacket." And the little old lady said, "Well, you don't want to change. I hear that. You want to stay in your pink jacket and your blue dress." And she looked at the other twin and said, "You want to know what others think before you are ready to decide to change."

And she looked at the two and she said to the first one, "Are you happy? And do you get what you want?" And the first twin looked down and tears came to her eyes and she said, "You know, I do everything I can think of to please. I spend a lot of time and effort, and yet I don't seem to know how to please and I do want to change." And the little voice inside said, "Yes, yes, change, change. You need to change." And the other twin looked at the lady and said crossly, "Change? I don't know how to change. I don't even know what would happen if I changed. I probably would hate myself in a pink jacket. No, I mean a blue jacket. I have a pink jacket. What do I mean? I don't know what I mean. I just feel disagreeable all the time."

And the little old lady said, "Maybe you do need to change." And so the second twin said sullenly, "Oh, what's the difference? Nothing's any good anyway. So, okay, I'll change." So she ripped off her pink jacket and she flung it at her twin. And the other twin took off her blue jacket and she handed it with a pleading look to the other. And so the first twin put on the pink jacket that matched her dress, and the other twin put on the blue jacket that matched her dress. And they changed. And what do you know, the second twin said to the first one, "Thank you for giving me the jacket that matches my dress." And the first twin said, "I'm glad I decided to ask for the jacket that matches my dress. I think that they got mixed up in the first place." And they smiled at each other for the first time in their lives, and the little old lady nodded and said, "Thank you for visiting me." And both twins smiled at her and said, "Thank you for the tea. Goodbye." And they walked out of the house, and do you know, from that moment on they started to agree with each other, and they stopped quarreling.

After the story, Trudy became more open to accepting her feelings, especially her anger. She gradually came to recognize her part in producing the unsatisfactory relationships she had always experienced. She joined a handball club and learned to hit hard. She liked to sing and discovered that she had a good voice, so she enrolled in a music school and studied voice. Eventually she joined a church choir. She became more assertive and gradually more responsible. She decided to leave her lover. Trudy still comes in for occasional "booster shots," as she calls these sessions. And she is taking charge of her life.

6

The Little Plum Tree

(A Story for a Client With Separation Anxiety Disorder)

Mrs. M. called to ask me to make an appointment for her daughter, Angela. I explained that Angela would have to make her own appointment with me. Mrs. M. replied that Angela would never agree to come to see me on her own. I asked if Angela would be willing to come in with Mrs. M. and then I could see them together. Mrs. M. sounded relieved and readily accepted the idea.

They arrived together, two remarkably pleasant, attractive women who looked more like sisters than like mother and daughter. Actually, Mrs. M. was only 18 years older than Angela, who had just celebrated her thirty-third birthday. Mrs. M. did most of the talking and answered all questions, whether addressed to her or to Angela. She explained that Angela had always been a delicate, sensitive child. No mother had ever had a daughter "sweeter, more considerate, more loving" than Angela. Perhaps Angela was too sensitive and unselfish for her own good. She and Angela had always been very close. There were times when Mrs. M. didn't think she could have "made it" if it hadn't been for little Angela.

Angela was a posthumous baby, born six months after her father's tragic death in a plane crash only five months after their wedding. At 18 years of age, Mrs. M. was a grieving young widow. Angela "saved her life." They were inseparable. Mrs. M. was both mother and father to her little daughter, and as Angela grew up, they became even closer, if that were possible.

The reason Mrs. M. wanted me to see Angela was that the doctors had "given up" on Angela. They said that they could find no physiological basis for Angela's condition and of late two different doctors had suggested psychotherapy for her. This upset Angela. She felt rejected and misunderstood by the doctors. She thought they were accusing her, without actually saying it in so many words, of faking her condition. Angela had been shedding tears about this for weeks.

Mrs. M. suggested that she see me alone to talk about Angela's condition. I explained that I thought seeing them together would be a better plan; since they were so close it would be a more direct and effective way to get to the heart of the difficulty.

In the sessions which followed, Angela sat quietly and placidly while Mrs. M. talked. She was attentive and nonverbally responsive to everything her mother said and did. She would nod with approval, and look sad or cheerful depending on the clues her mother provided. Mrs. M. proved to be unusually verbal. Angela had been a model baby and toddler. However, she had been quite timid and anxious around strangers and would cling to her mother whenever, for any reason, Mrs. M. had to leave her. She was fond of her grandmother but would not accept her as a babysitter. She would cry so piteously that Mrs. M. did not have the heart to go. So, she and Angela did everything together. Actually, it was lovely. They really got along so well together.

All through grade school and high school, Angela was impeded by poor health. She often would awaken with an earache or an upset stomach and was not able to be up and around until late afternoon. Once Mrs. M. enrolled Angela in a summer camp, but in little more than a week the camp director telephoned to report that Angela had spent the past week in the infirmary. Mrs. M. hurried to the camp and, when she saw *how sick Angela was, she took her home. Angela was clearly too frail for the strenuous camp activities. Later on, Angela dropped out of college as well. Then, although she was quite successful at getting clerical jobs, she soon would lose them because of absenteeism due to her delicate health. No, Angela had never seemed to want girl friends. Mother was her best friend. No, as yet, the "right boy friend" had not appeared on the scene.*

The crisis which precipitated Mrs. M.'s phone call to me was generated by her new plans to be remarried. She had met a dear, kind man at her church. One thing led to another, and she had fallen in love. He was a retired widower and "comfortably well-off." He wanted to spend their honeymoon on a round-the-world cruise. He would not hear of Angela's accompanying them. He was downright adamant about this. What's more, he insisted that Angela get her own apartment after the wedding.

Lately, Angela's health had deteriorated alarmingly. She felt so ill that she could not eat or sleep. She was losing a great deal of weight. She had terrible nightmares about horrible disasters befalling her mother and would awaken screaming and shaking in a cold sweat. Her mother would hold her in her arms until at last they both fell asleep. How could she possibly leave Angela? Angela wept silently as her mother tearfully spoke of her dilemma.

All along, in the preceding sessions, I had been teaching them to go into trance. It was at this point that the following story told itself.

O nce upon a time there was a beautiful plum tree which grew on the side of a hill in a lovely sunny place. It had a strong, slender trunk and its branches sprang from all sides like a lacy parasol of twigs and leaves. The sun came through them in filtered patterns, ever changing, ever moving, so that the little tree often seemed to be laughing. In the winter, all through the winter, the earth nourished the little plum tree and, although you couldn't see it, sap was rising to feed the little tree and to bring it strength. In the winter, when its branches were bare of leaves, and you could hardly tell that it had life, still life was stirring inside and its many roots were digging strong and firm into the rich earth that fed it.

As the winter passed, and the spring began to bring its gentle rain and sunshine, a miracle happened that transformed the little tree. Buds began to swell on all the twigs on every branch, and if you glanced quickly out of the corner of your eye you could see the buds growing and swelling each hour of the day because the time had come for the little plum tree to begin to bloom. One morning, the blossoms began to burst forth all over like a beautiful bouquet, and the little tree stood covered with fragrant flowers, trembling and floating and dancing in the spring air. Then there was a delightful gaiety, an air of celebration that shimmered around the whole little tree. It had reached yet another cycle in its wonderful round of cycles! The white blossoms increased and grew in brilliance. Then gradually they began to fade, to curl up, to fall gently floating to the earth as graceful in their descent as they had been in their blooming. Behind them they left little beginning fruits of the plum, deep red, shining and hard, which covered the tree on all its branches and twigs. And they were as beautiful in their own way as the blossoms had been. So the little tree, the little plum tree, began to fruit. Each day the plums grew larger, ever more and more mature, ripening in their turn in their beautiful cycle, coming to full ripeness. Then the birds came from everywhere and nested in the branches of the happy little plum tree. They ate plums and sang songs of thanks to the tree. Sometimes in their haste they would free a plum from its branch and it would fall and roll, full of mischievous bounce and energy, far from the trunk of the little plum tree and come to rest in a soft, warm hollow of the rich moist earth.

That is how it came to be, that is how it happened, that one day a little seed in the heart of the plum came to rest very deep in a hollow of the earth. And the grasses covered it, and the little plum wrinkled and dried, and at last it released the beautiful hard brown seed it held in its heart. The seed found a place in the earth and began to set forth its own roots, finding its nourishment independent of the plum tree, finding its own nourishment through its own roots, growing stronger, bigger, more complicated, reaching deeper and deeper into the rich and nourishing earth, taking its food, growing its own slender twiglike trunk and putting out its first tiny branches. So it grew, day by day, until the autumn came with its many changing rains and clouds and winds, and then the winter with its cold and silent sleep. The little plum tree still looked like a mere twig, but its roots grew strong and sturdy and in its turn it too took nourishment from the earth, just like the parent tree before it. It began to gather its own strength so that when spring comes, joyous in its freedom, it too will put forth blossoms and leaves and fruit in its own cycle, separate from the parent tree nearby.

I followed up the story with reinforcing sessions focused on "normalizing" change, cycles, and development. Mrs. M. vacillated about her wedding. Angela slowly became more cheerful. Spring gave way to summer and summer to autumn. When winter arrived, Mrs. M.'s fiance delivered an ultimatum. He set an arbitrary date. He made reservations for a world tour. He demanded a definite yes or no. With my support, Mrs. M. decided to say "yes."

Angela was hospitalized. I saw her daily when her mother departed. With frequent hypnotherapy sessions, Angela slowly began to attach herself to me. I was in weekly telephone contact with Mrs. M. As Angela gradually differentiated from her mother, she began to make significant changes. At the present time, she is sharing an apartment with two new friends she met in group therapy sessions. She is considering returning to school. She has made an appointment with a vocational guidance counselor to help her choose a field of interest.

Angela sees her mother and new stepfather frequently. Her initial daily telephone calls to her mother are spacing out considerably, as have her sessions with me. There are good indications that the new little plum tree "will put forth blossoms and leaves and fruit in its own cycle, separate from the parent tree nearby."

7

Secret Room

(A Story for a Client With
Passive-Aggressive Personality Disorder
Who Plays Schlemiel)

Michael was not sure he wanted to come to see me. He hemmed and hawed, saying a good friend suggested that he come . . . but he didn't know. A small-boned young man of 23, nice-looking, soft-spoken, he was hesitant about making eye contact. He mentioned that he stuttered when he was a child, and also had difficulty with learning to read. The reason, he said, his friend suggested that he seek "help" was that he seemed unable to relate intimately with anyone and was unsuccessful in either initiating or accepting a love relationship. Consequently, he felt depressed much of the time. Employed in a routine department store job selling men's clothing, he complained about being unappreciated and unrewarded. His boss bullied him. Even his mother, father and siblings were unsupportive and disapproving. Then, after minutes of silent inner struggle, he announced, "I'm gay."

Michael was slow to trust me. By playing dumb, he tried to mask his feelings of shame and inadequacy, as well as his fears of being punished by his family or his boss. His own expression for himself was "dumb blonde." Below the surface, his suppressed anger seethed. With his friends, he dodged accepting responsibility by acting out "schlemiel."

At first resistant to trance, he gradually relaxed enough to allow himself to be hypnotized. He began to trust me, and after some six months of treatment, mostly centered on self-esteem and trust, the following story told itself.

T his is a story about a little boy who was quite, quite little, and this little boy lived in a very pretty house. It was
a sunny, bright, cheerful house, and there were lots of friendly
people there, all his family. It was really quite cheerful, quite
pleasant, and quite enjoyable. All the rooms were full of light,
shining and pretty, and sparkling clean. And the little boy felt
very safe and very good except for one thing. When he was
very, very, very little, he had discovered a secret room in his
house. And that secret room seemed to be unknown to everyone except him. He was the only one who went there, and
he seemed to be the only one who knew about it. It was a small
room, a dark room, and he was afraid to let anyone know about
his secret room because he thought maybe he had just made
it up and no one would believe him. Or it could be they all
knew something about it that he didn't know and that they
didn't want to tell him. Or that there was some reason that
everyone knew but him. And so he never let on to anyone
about his secret room. He would go there and he would close
the door, and shut himself in, and sometimes he would scare
himself in there, all the time trying to puzzle out the secret
of the room that everyone either didn't know was there . . . but
him, or else pretended they didn't know was there.

And it came to be that as the days passed, he spent more
and more time in his secret room and less and less time in the
sunny, cheerful rooms outside with the others. And sometimes
when he was in his room, his little secret room, he would be
afraid he would get locked in and not be able to get out again,
and this would frighten him very much. At those times he
would come out of his room in a great hurry, and for a while
he would make himself very busy joining with the others and
doing whatever it was that they were doing and pretending
that there was no secret room in his house. But sooner or later

he always went back. And soon he would go there more and more often. He lost his cheerfulness and his happiness, and he began to feel very lonely because, when he spent so much time in his secret room, he had to interrupt the games that he played with the others. Sometimes even right in the middle of hearing a story, he felt he had to stop, make up an excuse, and run to his secret room. Sometimes he noticed that when he was in there he began to confuse himself, and he thought, "Why am I confusing myself?"

One day as he was sitting there asking himself, "Why am I confusing myself?" he heard a little voice that came out of the corner of the room, and the little voice said, "Dummy . . . you confuse yourself when you put on that dunce cap." And the little boy said, "What dunce cap?" The little voice said, "Reach up and feel it." He reached up and sure enough, he felt a tall pointed dunce cap. Oh, he was so angry! He stamped his feet and tore the dunce cap off and threw it on the floor. The little voice in the corner said, "He, he, he . . . the next time you come in, you'll do the same thing, dummy, because every time you come in, the first thing you do is you put on your dunce cap." And the little boy said, "Go away. I don't want to talk to you. Go away." Then he rushed out of the secret room and slammed the door. Outside the room he looked all around, frightened that someone had heard him slam the door and might find out about the secret room — or worse, know that he knew about the secret room.

And so the days passed. And more and more, right in the middle of being hugged, or right in the middle of really enjoying himself, right in the middle of enjoying new friends and doing all the things he really liked doing, he would have to stop himself, make an excuse, and run back to shut himself up in his little room. Soon, whenever he was away from the room, he began to worry that someone would find out about his room. And he told himself, "Then I won't have it all to myself anymore, and what they'll do is laugh at me and make a fool of me like that horrible little voice in the corner." So more and more often he went into his room, his little dark room, and locked himself in. And he thought, "It is my secret," and the little voice in the corner said, "He, he, he . . . you have your dunce cap on again." And the little boy would take the dunce cap off and think about tearing it up, but he never could do it. He grew afraid as he thought, "Pretty soon I'll be spend-ing all of my time in my little room, alone. I seem to be there more and more often now. Just last week, I met such a neat kid down the block, and I would like to be his friend, but I don't have time anymore. I seem to have to be in my little room longer and longer." And he looked downcast and felt so unhappy. He was so, so very unhappy. He didn't know what to do.

One day, when he had just come out of his secret room, just before he closed the door, he noticed that someone was sitting beside the door. So he hastily closed the door. And then he tried to pretend that he was just walking around. He smiled and he said, "Hello, who are you?" He saw, sitting there, a very old person. The old person was smiling at him. And the old person said, "I saw your room." Oh, oh, oh, the little boy felt terrified, and he began to shake. "Oh, no," he said, "there is no room. There is no room. No, no room." But the old per-son said, "It's a secret room, isn't it?" And the little boy said, "No . . . no room. There is no room." The old person smiled and said, "But I saw it. And you spend a lot of time in there, don't you?" The little boy began to cry and nod his head. And the old person said, "When you go in, there is a hat you put on, isn't there?" And the little boy said, "How do you know?"

And the old person said, "I know because I have known other little boys, and they also have secret rooms, and when they go in, they also put on hats so they can confuse themselves, and they also think that no one else has a secret room or a secret, and they are afraid. . . . And there's a voice that talks to you in there, isn't there?" And the little boy nodded miserably. The old person said, "And the little voice calls you a dunce, right?" And the little boy really began to sob, as he said, "Oh, please, please, tell me what to do. I don't know what to do." And the old person said, "Yes, you do. Yes, you do." "No, I don't. No, I don't," said the little boy, and the old person said, "You can listen for other voices." And the little boy said, "I don't know how to do that." The old person said, "Next time you go in, leave the door open." "OOOH, I couldn't do that . . ," said the little boy. "If I leave the door open, then other people will know I have a secret room." And the wise old person nodded and said, "And then it won't be secret anymore." And the little boy said, "Yes." And the old person said, "And then . . . ?" "Well, I don't know," said the little boy. So the old person said, "I will go with you. Will you go with me and together we'll leave the door open?"

The little boy trembled and shook with fright, but he took the old gnarled hand extended to him. And together they went into the little secret dark room. And they left the door ajar. With the light shining into the room, the little boy looked around and saw that there were many, many creatures in there. They looked very friendly. And he saw with surprise and delight that they all looked very much like him. "Oh," he said to the old person, "look at all these little friends, and they all look like me." And the old person nodded and smiled. He said, "Would you like to speak to them?" "Well, I don't know," said the little boy. And the little voices all said in a chorus, "Oh, yes, please speak to us." But the other voice in the corner said, "Dummy, dummy, put on your hat. Quick, put on your hat so you'll be confused." And the other voices said, "No, no, no, don't do it. Don't listen to him, listen to us."

And so they began to talk to him, and they said, "You made this room a secret because you didn't let any light in." And the wise old person nodded. The little boy said, "Well, I've left the door open now." "Yes, yes," they said, "look around," and he looked around and saw that there were other doors, and he saw that there were windows, and the little friends said, "Open them, open them," and so he went to the windows and he opened one. When he looked through it, he saw a wonderful, wonderful scene—it was a beautiful countryside. They said, "Open more . . . open more." And he opened another, and he saw a lovely room filled with friendly people. And they said, "Open another one . . . open another one!" They were all excited and happy for him. And so he opened another, and there, he saw a beautiful library, and it was full of books and records, and there were people singing and dancing. Others were reading and learning, and then to his astonishment, he found door after door, and he saw that his secret room really had no walls, but was all doors and windows. He went from one to another, leaving them open, and he found that HE COULD GO FROM HIS SECRET ROOM INTO ANY PLACE HE CHOSE.

He turned to the old person and said, "Oh, what a magical world." And the old person nodded and said, "Yes, that is the secret you wouldn't let yourself know. You have all these doors, and you can open them to a wonderful world." The little boy looked all around and saw that his secret room was full of light and windows and open doors. He walked out, and he said to his family, "I want you to meet my new friend . . . my old . . . ," but when he turned, his old friend was waving good-bye and saying, "You don't need me anymore." So the little boy turned to share his secret with his family and invited them to come into his secret room, which was no longer a secret, and there he introduced all his new friends.

After the story, changes began to occur. Michael studied for and passed a state real estate agent's licensing exam with flying colors, and joined a real estate firm. He volunteered to serve on the Gay Hot-Line. He became active in the Gay Rights movement. His circle of friends expanded rapidly. He discovered that many people respected him! Little more than a year later he invited a lover to share his apartment. When I last heard, Michael had bought a condominium and was living happily with Randy.

8

The Little Crab

(A Story for a Client
With Oppositional Disorder)

Mrs. J. called for an appointment for her 12-year-old son, Dennis. I asked her to come with him. During this phone call she said she was "at the end of her rope" because Dennis was in so much trouble at school.

Mrs. J., a single parent, and Dennis, an only child, arrived on schedule. Mrs. J. was in her mid-thirties. She proved to be articulate, business-like and emphatic. It was only when she talked about her son that her voice took on a slight whine. Slender, meticulously dressed and coiffed, with every bleached hair in place, she described herself as a devoted mother who carried the burden of rearing her son alone. She was also an "achiever" who had worked her way up from a job as a trained nurse to an impressive administrative position in a major hospital. She described long, hard hours of work. She is working harder than ever now. Up until the last year, Dennis had been a source of pride to her that "made it all worthwhile."

Dennis slouched in his chair, looking at the ceiling, jiggling his Nike-clad foot which rested on the opposite thigh. A good-looking boy, he was well-built, even manly. He appeared to be a fine, healthy 12-year-old. As his mother talked, Dennis shifted around restlessly in his chair. Without pausing, she interjected, "Sit up straight, Dennis," and continued her narrative without missing a beat. When she gestured to him, signaling him to tuck in his shirttails, Dennis made a token move to do so, leaving half still hanging out. In a few moments, still talking, she signaled him to tuck in that other half. After a minute or two he complied. Without a pause, she went on describing him as an unusually bright, good baby and a dear little boy — so handsome, so helpful, so considerate — a perfect little gentleman. Everyone complimented her on having such an exemplary child. Dennis' ears were turning a hot red. She continued that there were nothing but good reports from school, from his piano teacher, from Sunday school class, from Cub Scouts, from his swimming instructor, and from the church where he was an altar boy. But starting about a year ago, Dennis began to have trouble.

Whenever I addressed a question to Dennis, Mrs. J. would answer for him. If I held up my hand to stop her, and Dennis started to talk, she would interrupt and take over. In ensuing sessions, she described her ex-husband, a well-known, successful stockbroker, as an alcoholic. Dennis studied the carpet between his feet. Yes, he did pay for Dennis' private school and did provide some child support. It was the school that was making all the trouble now. It seemed that Dennis was just fine at home. But she kept getting reports about his failure to live up to his potential, even failing to turn in homework assignments although she supervised his studies every night. Teachers in all his classes, except physical education, complained that he refused to observe classroom rules, was inattentive, "talked back" to instructors and even to the headmaster in whose office he was spending more and more of his school time. They claimed that he disrupted the class by throwing spitballs (Dennis protested that the other kids started it), passing notes, making facetious comments, and putting graffiti on the blackboard. He was having trouble with his peer group as well. There were several big boys in the class who "picked on" Dennis. Often they succeeded in provoking him into losing his temper and starting a fight.

Then Mrs. J. confided that she felt very uncomfortable with

the headmaster and the teachers. She thought they were criticizing her. She never had felt really comfortable with the other mothers and rarely participated in parent-teacher activities. She described the parents of the school children as being rich and very social. The mothers did not have to work. She thought they looked down on her because she was divorced and had a job. Mrs. J. felt like an outsider.

Whenever Dennis did talk, which was not very often and usually in short bursts between long squirming silences, he described his teachers as being unreasonable and picking on him. He professed to be mystified by their complaints. He thought they disliked him and were "pushing him around." He said that when he asked for help with his homework they accused him of arguing and being stubborn. The headmaster took the teachers' side. The big boys who provoked him into fighting rages were bullies who were probably jealous because he was a pretty good soccer player and the best pitcher on the softball team. Looking up, with a rebellious scowl, he said they kept calling him "Dennis the Menace" in high, falsetto voices. He muttered that he wanted to be called "Butch" like his dad. It was at this point in treatment that the following story was told.

A s you follow a winding path, you come to the house of a storyteller. And you love stories, so you go into the house where sits a very aged storyteller who greets you and asks you to sit down, please. She says that she has a special story for you today. She asks if you would like to hear it, and you say, "Oh, yes, thank you."

And the story begins about once upon a time . . . there was a little baby crab by the ocean, and this little crab would stick its head out of its little house in the sand early in the morning, and would look this way and that way fearfully, and then go back into its hole. It repeated this strange behavior until it got so very hungry that at last it had to come out. Very tentatively, very slowly, and very fearfully, the little crab came out of its hole in the sand. And it looked this way and that way and this way and that way. When it saw no danger, it began to look for food. And believe it or not, right there ahead of it, near the water's edge, it spotted a succulent breakfast. And so the little crab thought it would scamper quickly over there. But a strange thing happened. When it meant to go forward, it found itself going backwards. Oh, what a terrible shock that whenever the little crab wanted to go forward, its legs would carry it backwards. This happened over and over until the little crab began to cry very pitifully. It sat in the sand, and felt very hungry, but it couldn't go where it wanted to go because every time it tried to go forward, it went backward instead. What it didn't know was that that's the way all crabs move.

Suddenly it heard a voice, a deep voice, and the little crab looked around with great fear. What it saw standing in front of it was a big old crab looking down at the baby crab and saying, "Now, what's the trouble, little crab?" The little crab said, "Oh, my, every time I want to go forward to get my breakfast, and I'm so hungry, every time I do that I go backwards." "Ho, ho, ho," said the crab, "that's very funny because that's what you're supposed to do." And the little crab said, "What do you mean?" "Well," said the big old crab, "everybody knows that crabs go backwards, and sometimes sideways when they want to get from here to there. That's why your eyes can see in back of you." "Oh," said the little crab. "I didn't know that." "Just look at me," said the old crab, and he scampered sideways, this way very fast, and then reversed and went sideways the other way very fast, and the little crab began to smile and decided to try doing it too. Sure enough, the little crab could scoot sideways in one direction and then sideways in another, and things began to seem better because the little crab thought, "Ah, if in the corner of my eye I see something there to one side, I can scoot over there as fast as anything . . . sideways." The old crab said, "Try it."

And sure enough, over there to the right, the little crab, without even appearing to be looking in that direction, saw a succulent breakfast. And zing, as fast as the twinkling of an eye, it scooted sideways and grabbed its breakfast before the baby breakfast knew what happened. "Oh," said the little crab, "how useful for me that when I seem to be pointing forward I scoot sideways. That is a wonderful thing to be able to do!" "And now," said the big crab, "watch me." And while the big crab seemed to be pointing toward the little crab, zing, in the flash of an eye, the big crab had gone backwards ever so far, ever so fast, and snapped up a tasty morsel of food. Oh, the little crab laughed with joy and then directed its eyes backwards in oh-so-clever a way. It could see in back of itself without seeming to be looking and without making the slightest sign that it was going to move back. In a flash, it had scooted backwards, ever so far, and snatched up another morsel of breakfast.

"There," said the big old crab, "now you know how useful it is to have ways of moving yourself that are natural to you. You don't go forward like many other creatures. You can go sideways and backwards faster than most creatures can go forward and that's because you are a little crab. Now, were you a fish, that would not be useful for you. Were you a bird, that probably wouldn't work. But for a little crab on the beach it's exactly suitable." And the little crab said, "Oh, thank you, thank you very much. This is the happiest day of my life." And the old wise crab said, "Yes, and it is also the first day of the rest of your life so enjoy yourself, little crab." And the little crab said, "Oh, I will. I really will." For the rest of the day it practiced scooting backwards ever so fast, and sideways in each direction ever so fast, and each time felt more joyous.

That is the end of the story. Now you thank the old story-teller, and you go out of the house, and taking your own good time you follow the winding path in your own way, and you come back here.

Both mother and son went into trance during the story, but I directed my voice primarily to Dennis. After the story he began to respond more openly to me. He enjoyed going into trance and liked stories, so I told many more after that. However, it was this initial story which served as an important turning point in the treatment. Dennis clearly heard the metaphoric permission to accept himself. Mrs. J. heard it too.

In following sessions Dennis' father joined us from time to time. Mr. J. was, in fact, a recovering alcoholic. He was also an "outdoors man." (Mrs. J. described him as "macho.") He undertook to teach his son to fish and hunt. He played catch and practiced shooting baskets with him. Dennis was a natural athlete so we encouraged and praised his athletic accomplishments. When he enrolled in a public junior high school near his house, his peer group problems were resolved. Now his friends lived nearby so he became "one of the boys" after school, which carried over into the classroom as well. Den-

nis was tutored during the summer before enrolling in his new school. He got along well with his young college student tutor, and he decided to start new classes "with a clean slate." He introduced himself as "Butch."

Mrs. J. still comes in for sessions with me. She is working on issues in which Dennis is not primarily involved. Butch has been doing quite well.

9

The Narcissus Bulb

(A Story for a Client in
Treatment for Depressive Neurosis)

Linda was referred to me by her physician. He suggested psychotherapy since he could find no physiological basis for her dysfunction. On her first visit I observed a somewhat overweight woman in her thirties. She spoke in a flat monotone, slowly and tonelessly. She gazed past my left shoulder or down at the floor, never once meeting my eyes as she hugged her arms across her chest. Her hair was carelessly combed and rather stringy. She wore no cosmetics and her clothes were nondescript, too short and a little too tight. She expressed pessimism about seeing a therapist. She thought hypnotherapy was "far out" and doubted that she could be hypnotized.

She went on to say that when she was in her early twenties she had been married and divorced after only two years. She thought she never should have married. She just didn't have what it takes to be a "good wife." When I asked what she thought it takes to be a good wife, she replied that her ex-husband got tired of her. He told her he was fed-up with her whining and her negativity. So then, what good was hypnotherapy since she was a "total failure with no possibilities left" for her? All her friends had let her down. Even her own mother refused to help her anymore. The world was cold and indifferent, dog-eat-dog, and she just wanted to give up.

Linda described herself as a "false alarm," lots of promise but with nothing actually delivered. In the music department at the University she had been considered a highly promising mezzo-soprano. But when she applied for admittance to the really top-rated New York and New England music schools for graduate training, she was turned down. She had gone east anyway, hoping to be accepted as a private student by a certain well-known ex-Metropolitan Opera star, but she remained on a waiting list and never made it. She supported herself by working as a waitress. She did get a little work as a "voice" on radio. She also sang at various functions, but rarely was paid. People used her. No one was willing to help her. She lived in a basement "cubbyhole." She borrowed from friends and owed money to everyone. She didn't see how she could possibly get out of debt ever again. One by one her friends became quarrelsome and turned against her. She went from bad to worse until she would find herself bursting into tears at her job in the restaurant while waiting on tables. She would be walking down the street and discover that tears were rolling down her face. Finally, when the friend who had sublet the little basement room to her returned to the city, she had no place to go. She came back to her hometown. Her mother took her in but she felt miserable there. She and her mother never had "hit it off." They screamed at each other constantly. Her doctor thought that perhaps I could help her. So here she is — at "the end of the road."

Linda went into trance easily and we started our work with brief episodes focused on self-esteem. She agreed to listen nightly to the tape I made for her.* I reframed despair as a period of lying fallow and gathering strength. Quite early in the course of treatment, the following story appeared.

---

*See the Introduction, p. 7.

This is a story about little plants who need the dark. Now, isn't that an interesting thing that there should be a plant that really needs the dark, because everyone knows that plants need light and sunlight and daylight in order to grow and develop and bloom. They need to come out of the dark earth where their roots are held and to rise out of the darkness and grow. But these are special plants because they grow from bulbs. So this story is about little plants that need the dark.

Once upon a time, there was a little girl who went to a flower store. There she saw a bin full of what looked like strange onions. They were very dry and dark brown and they really did not look as though they would be very good to eat. As a matter of fact, they looked quite dead. So she asked the storekeeper, "What are those?" And the storekeeper came over—he was a kindly old man—and explained to her that what she was looking at were narcissus bulbs. "Oh," she said, "I know the story of Narcissus. Narcissus was the young god who looked into the pool and saw the image of himself, and fell instantly in love with the beautiful creature he saw there." And the storekeeper said, "What an interesting story." "Oh, yes," she said, "that's Greek."

"Well," he said, "what an intelligent and well-read little girl you are to know such a beautiful story about Narcissus. For that reason, because I think you are so bright, I'm going to give you one of these bulbs." "Oh, thank you," she said. "I will go and plant it right away." But he said, "Wait, this bulb needs special treatment. I will tell you what you must do. This bulb needs darkness." She said, "Darkness?" "Oh, yes, because if it gets into the light before it is ready, it will not develop a deep enough root system, and so its stem and its leaves will be weak and pale and it might not even come to flower. So you must put it in this sandy loam which I will give you in this little pot, and there will be pebbles and you will keep water around the little bulb, which then must stay in a dark place, perhaps a little closet, or a small cupboard, until one day when you peek in, you will see a small, bright, green shoot which will come right out of the top of this bulb. Now look carefully, this is the top and there at the bottom are the little beginning roots. When you see that shoot grow several inches in the dark, then you will take it out into the light and then you will see a miracle as lovely as the story of Narcissus."

So the little girl ran home with her bulb and her little pot of pebbles and loam. As soon as she arrived she carefully put the little bulb in the pot and covered it over with pebbles. Then she found a safe, cool place in a closet and she put it there. Every day she peeked in to see if something had happened, and for many days she couldn't see that anything had happened. And she became very impatient after a while, thinking, "Oh, this little plant is never going to do anything in the dark." But she remembered what the wise old storekeeper had told her and she thought, "Well, I will keep it in the dark a little longer, just a little longer." And each day she said, "Well, a few more days," but all the time her heart grew heavier because she thought, "Oh, it isn't true that anything can grow in the dark, and he was probably teasing me. Everyone knows that you have to have sunshine and light to grow."

And so she began to doubt and doubt and she felt anxious until she herself looked as though she needed some sunshine and some light because she grew pale and sad. Then one day, she opened the closet door and her face lit up with joy because she saw peeking through the pebbles the tiniest, lightest, most tender green shoot that anyone could imagine. "Oh, Narcissus," she said. "How beautiful you are!" And she smiled with joy and felt her heart fill with love and hope and she told herself, "You must be patient. Remember? He said that it must stay in the dark until it develops a strong root system and that is natural for it, and when the green shoot is sturdy and strong because enough roots have been grown, then I can take my beautiful Narcissus plant into the light."

And every day, filled with joy, she would open the closet door to look, and sure enough, every day the green shoot was stronger and taller, until one day, she thought, surely that is the right height because it was a full three inches above the pebbles. Gently, gently, she took it out into the light. Oh, she thought, sunlight would be too strong for this so first I will just bring it into daylight. And she was so happy because she could look at it and see her beautiful Narcissus every day for longer and longer hours. And she noticed that it grew strong and tall and slender and graceful. It looked so joyous and healthy that she thought, "I can see Narcissus smiling at me!" And she smiled back with pleasure and happiness to see this beautiful plant that grew so tall and so healthy and so strong.

Then one day she saw a marvelous sight. She saw thrusting out of the leaves on the stem the most lovely, perfect bud. "Oh," she said, "how lovely. I will move my plant a little nearer to the sunshine, and I will watch closely now because I believe that my Narcissus is about to bloom." And sure enough, the next day, she saw the first little petal of the flower emerge. And the next day three more. And the next day she saw the beautiful, lovely bells that opened and she was filled with joy, understanding that Narcissus was special and needed the dark to grow roots and strength and that once its strength and roots were developed, this lovely plant could flourish in the daylight and that it needed the daylight to come to flower and fulfill its cycle. And there it stood, beautiful, fresh and blooming, the first to bloom of all the plants who were waiting for a later time and didn't need the darkness as Narcissus did. And the little girl said, "Of all the plants and flowers, you are the one I love most." And it seemed to her almost as though the plant responded. And so, from then on the little girl understood the uses of darkness and light, and that both are needed for some plants.

After the story, Linda responded to our work with signs of new hopefulness. Her energy seemed renewed, and she roused herself from her lethargy enough to take long walks several times a week. She discovered a library nearby and spent hours there, away from her mother. At last, she began to practice her singing again. Her mother enjoyed Linda's songs!

After several months, Linda announced that she had a job as a waitress in an all-night restaurant on the riverfront. She felt enthusiastic because it was a favorite meeting place for jazz musicians to gather after their work to "jam" in the early morning hours. Linda had been waitressing there only for three weeks when one of the groups heard her sing and invited her to "jam" with them. Soon she was singing with several different groups every night whenever the restaurant business slacked off. Then one night a group talked about plans to cut a record, and they asked Linda to join them.

At present our sessions have spaced out to once a month. She is actively seeking "spot" employment with local radio stations. Her new musician friends have recommended her for voice dubbing assignments in commercials. She is making plans to move out of her mother's house to her own apartment.

10

All the Creatures in the Forest

(A Story for a Client With
a Gender Identity Disorder)

*H*enry was exceptionally handsome, tall and slender, with a beautiful, strong-featured, sensitive face. He moved with a natural grace. And although he spoke quietly and was barely audible, his resonant voice was richly baritone.

His story unfolded slowly, in bits and pieces, fits and starts. Soon to turn 20 years of age, he was a student in a local ballet dance studio. He had difficulty disciplining his body, and hated his muscularity and what he thought was the male inflexibility of his ankles, wrists and pelvis. He longed to dance the roles of the ballerinas. He detested the male roles of "leaping and strutting." In fact, he found his male body "disgusting." Actually, he said, he felt like a female "inside"—always had, as far back as he could remember.

He had been reading about operations which changed males into females. Did I think that might be a possibility for him?

We began hypnotherapy. During one early trance session, Henry introduced me to "Henrietta." Henrietta told me that she was five years old. She had many friends, little girls in her neighborhood who played with her. Henrietta was cheerful and self-confident. Henrietta thought little boys were "nasty."

As we explored his history, Henry talked about his parents and his two older sisters. His mother divorced his father when Henry was almost two years old. He scarcely knew his father, except through his mother's scornful descriptions of a "weakling," a "loser," who thought his "disgusting penis" was the most important thing in the world, a sufficient excuse for his lazy, ne'er-do-well habits.

Among countless other details, Henry recalled an episode which took place when he was quite little. His mother came into his room and saw him masturbating. She slapped his hands hard and screamed, "Disgusting, nasty, and if you keep on doing that it will shrivel up and fall off!!" It seems that Henry's mother screamed often, especially when she was drinking. Henry was afraid of her, but he also loved her and longed for her approval. He felt certain that she loved his sisters more than she loved him. He used to put on his sisters' clothes and pretend to be a girl. They all would make fun of him. Even now, whenever he had the chance, he would dress up in his mother's clothes. Only now he did it in secret.

Men often made sexual overtures to him, but he disliked homosexual males, and after several experiments, he now avoided them. What he longed for was female companionship. He felt like them inside, and passionately wished to be one of them. He felt ugly. He felt different from everyone else — not fitting in anywhere — an outsider. He felt lonely.

At this point the following story appeared.

O nce upon a time in a leafy forest, there were all manner of little creatures — little furry creatures, little feathered creatures, little scaly creatures — and, although they were different from each other, they all felt pretty good about themselves because they were surrounded by mothers and fathers, sisters and brothers, each all feathered like them, or furred like them, or scaly like them. So they felt very comfortable about themselves. Their mothers and fathers helped to make them feel comfortable about themselves. And not one ever thought, "It's strange that I have scales and my friend over there is furry," because they took it for granted that some of them would be furry, and some of them would have scales, and some of them would have feathers. They all lived together quite contented and quite pleased with themselves so that life was pleasant, and day followed day in a very cheerful and relaxed fashion.

If a newcomer came, wearing his scales, and stopped in astonishment to see a furry creature, and said, "What is the matter with you? What has happened to your scales? You are really strange-looking with that funny fur all over you when you should have scales," the furry little fellow would say, "Why, you are the one who is silly. Do you think everyone has scales? Not at all. Not at all. Look around. Lots of us do have scales. But we are all okay even though we are different." "Oh," said the scaly newcomer, looking around, "I guess I just never saw anyone with fur before. So I guess I was surprised. And I haven't ever seen anyone with feathers either, so I think I was surprised, but now I see what you mean."

When first he had seen the furry creatures, although he had said, "What's the matter with you?" inside he was thinking, "Oh, what could be the matter with me that I have these smooth and shiny scales when that creature over there is all soft and furry." But when he understood that they were different from him, and that it was okay, then he grew cheerful, forgot about it, and began to play with all the other little creatures.

One day, an entirely different young creature came into the forest. This one didn't fly in the air, and didn't walk on four legs, and had no scales, and no feathers, and very little fur. This one was a very, very strange creature. This one walked on two legs and had a naked skin and had a patch of fur on top in the strangest way. Most of this creature was entirely without scales or feathers or fur. What a strange-looking creature! All the little creatures stopped whatever they were doing and stared. There was silence in the forest. Scaly ones, and the ones with fur, and the feathered ones stopped their playing, and stopped their chatter.

The newcomer looked around, then a surprising thing happened. From the tips of its two feet that it stood upon, red color began to rise up its legs, then up its body and down its arms to its fingertips, then up its neck until finally its whole face and body were flaming red. Then it spoke, "What is the matter? Why are all you strange creatures looking at me?" He said, "Really, it is you who are strange. Some of you are all covered with scales, and some of you are all covered with fur, and some of you have feathers from tip to tip. You are strange. Where I come from, people have skin, and they have hair in several places." He said, "But then, I have never seen myself. I saw my brothers and sisters, but maybe. . . ," he thought with horror, " . . . maybe I AM strange. Maybe I don't look like anyone else in the whole world. Maybe I just think I look like my brothers."

And the newcomer sat down on the ground. Tears began to roll down his bare cheeks. When this happened, all the other little creatures formed a circle around him and felt very sorry for him. They said, "You are strange, and we don't know where you come from or what manner of creature you are, but we will help you grow scales, or feathers or fur. Which do you want?" The new little person said, "I don't want scales. I mean no offense to you," he said looking around at the scaly creatures, "but I wouldn't like scales for me." And he looked at the feathered creatures and said, "I wouldn't want feathers

for me either, although it might be nice to fly." He thought
about that for a moment, then shook his head and said no.
"I really don't want that either. I don't mean to insult you, but
I really don't want any feathers." And he said to the furry
creatures, "Well, it might be nice to have fur, but I am used
to having it only on the top of my head, and a few other special
places." And quickly he felt to make sure he had it. "And I
really would like it just where I have it and not in any other
place. But maybe," he thought in his heart, "I'm wrong." So
the others said, "You do look very strange, but if you would
like to see what you look like, we'll take you to the pond, and
you can see yourself in there. Then you can decide if you want
to stay the way you are or whether you want to be like one
of us."

The newcomer was afraid to look into the water because
he was afraid of what he might see, afraid that he did not really
look like all the other creatures back there where he came
from. Afraid he would find that he was some kind of strange
creature unlike anyone else in the world. The others reassured
him and encouraged him, and cheered him on. And when he
looked around, he felt better because all at once he realized
that they had stopped pointing, had stopped being enemies,
and that they were now friendly, encouraging him and taking care of him. So he went along with them.

When they approached the pond he looked into the water
very timidly. Then he smiled at his image, because he saw that
he did indeed look like all the creatures back home, and not
only that, but that he looked as beautiful as the most beautiful
he remembered. He looked and he looked and he thought,
"I am very beautiful, and I am a 'he'; and even though I don't
have scales and I don't have fur and I don't have feathers, and
even though what I have is distributed in a very strange way,
I think I am beautiful." And so he turned to his new friends

and said, "Thank you for showing me myself and thank you for letting me see that I am beautiful even though I am different from you." So from that moment on, he played with his new friends and quite soon they forgot that he didn't have fur or feathers or scales like them, and he forgot that they had fur and scales and feathers unlike him. And so they all lived very happily together in the forest. All of the creatures realized that they were much more alike, each to the other, than they were different.

After the story, Henry began to assess himself in a more realistic frame of reference. For example, he remarked at the following session that he thought he would probably turn out to be a "very peculiar-looking woman." Over six feet tall, large-featured and broad-shouldered, he began to doubt that he could succeed as a ballerina.

The importance of this particular story in his treatment stemmed solely from his accomplishment of the first "break-through." There were many more episodes and more stories which followed. A great deal of work was still needed. Henry's sessions with me continued off and on for more than three years and I still see him at six-month intervals. At this point he has begun to socialize as a male. I believe that he will sooner or later seek out a female mate.

11

The Weathervane

(A Story for
Dependent Personality Disorder)

Margo presented herself attractively. She was trim and carefully groomed. Her clothes were fashionable in a subtle, played-down way that evoked a second look. She smiled engagingly and laughed readily. She almost apologized for having problems and listened eagerly to everything I said. Her manner was deferential and subtly seductive.

Margo was 30 years old at the time, married for six years and "in love" with her husband. They had two sons, five and three years of age. She worked for a well-known national distributor of cheese products in a responsible position as vice president in charge of Midwest distribution. Her job necessitated a great deal of traveling and she thought that her difficulty centered on her fear of flying. If the flight was longer than one hour, Margo became immobilized with fear. She postponed mandatory business meetings or arranged time-consuming alternative means of travel, often detouring in order to cut flight times down into hour-long segments. Her boss, who had acted as her mentor since the very beginning of her business career, was becoming impatient with her, threatening to replace her with someone willing to expand operations and to advance in the organization, which meant assuming responsibility for larger territories. She both respected and feared her boss. She didn't think she could manage without his support and guidance.

Margo responded quickly to hypnosis, and as we began to work in weekly sessions, she described her family as "very close." She spoke of her husband as "loving and supportive," her children as "bright and sweet" and mother as "wonderful." She didn't think she could possibly manage without her mother, who lived in their house with them. Her father died when she was 15 and her older sister was 18. Her regret was that she felt that she scarcely knew him. It seems that he was a hard-driving man, dedicated to his career, who was often away from home and who usually "had to" bring work home with him on the brief occasions when he did join the family. It was her mother who was the center of their household. And it was her mother who now provided the anchor for Margo in her marriage by holding down the fort while Margo worked, mothering her grandsons, and looking after the household. Her "loving mother" guided them all with her experience and wisdom. How did her husband and her mother get along? Well, her husband really never got along very well with his own mother, so "naturally" he would sometimes "back talk" his mother-in-law, but Margo, who loved them both, was adept at peacemaking.

Soon another aspect of Margo's difficulties began to emerge. She told me that during her adolescence she had suffered from an acne condition. She felt horribly self-conscious and spent hours treating her skin. She dreaded going out among strangers. She still felt self-conscious about her acne scars, which she was certain were disfiguring to her. I scanned her face but could not see any scars. Even now, she continued, she anxiously examined her face every morning, and whenever a pimple appeared on her skin she would burst into tears and have a tantrum. She felt embarrassed about this behavior, especially because her husband was becoming impatient, her mother very upset, and her children frightened. She was afraid of losing her looks, of becoming unattractive. She had always, all her life, most of all wanted to please and to be accepted.

Finally she confessed, most hesitantly, that her wish to please and be accepted led her to behave in ways that made her feel ashamed. It seems that she could not resist flirting with men she met in the course of doing her job, especially when she was out of town and alone too much. She described herself as a kind of female counterpart to a sailor with a girl in every port. She had a man in almost every town in her territory. She found it very exciting and dangerous, but afterwards she always felt miserably guilty and afraid. She truly loved her husband, loved her family. What could be wrong with her?

Two months passed and Margo continued to be cooperative and appeared eager to work for change, but no changes were apparent. It was at this point that the following story emerged.

O nce upon a time, there was a little weathervane that lived on the top of a very, very handsome barn. And as it looked around the farmyard, it could see all manner of creatures, all manner of different beings. There were milkmaids, rosy, plump and silly. There were all kinds of animals — cows mooing, returning to the barn with full udders, pigs oinking, fat and clever with their little beady eyes and sly smiles, hysterical chickens running this way and that . . . even rabbits hopping and twitching and wiggling their noses. All kinds — kittens, and cats, and dogs, and horses — and as the little weathervane looked at this scene, it thought, "If I could be one of them, how would I be? How would I want to be now? Would I want to be one of the big rough farmers striding about? How would

I have to be then for the others to love me?" And the little weathervane couldn't answer the question. Then it thought how it would be if it were a pig, or how it would feel to be a cow, or how it would have to behave to be a milkmaid, and each behavior it thought about was so different from how it would have to behave if it were something else that the little weathervane seemed to be confused most of the time. It would whirl this way, and then it would stop and turn all the way around and whirl the other way. It whirled this way, and it whirled that way until it was completely dizzy from whirling around. And it grew sad because it couldn't decide how to be.

One morning, there was a soft warm breeze blowing. The breeze came up and said, "Good morning, weathervane." And the little weathervane replied, "Well, good morning. What's your name?" And the little breeze said, "I'm the south wind, and when I blow, when I blow, you point straight that way," and she blew a warm puff. Sure enough, he turned and pointed that way. Then she laughed, and she left the little weathervane, who thought, "Well, I can just keep pointing the way the south wind blows, and that feels very good. but still, I'm not sure . . . is that going to be pleasing to everyone? Or will there be people who don't like the south wind? Oh, my, I wish I could decide."

About noontime, there came another voice and a big puff of wind. The little weathervane turned saying, "And who are you?" The wind said, "I am the west wind. I blow strong and dry, and where I blow, I bring change." The little weathervane said, "Oh, you are strong," and it felt itself turning around and going in an altogether different direction in spite of itself. Then it thought, "Even if I tried to face where the south wind blew, I wouldn't be able to. I seem to go whichever way the wind blows, and I'm not sure I like that."

Just then there came another voice. It was gruff, and it was strong, and it was angry, and it said, "I am the north wind, and you will point and face the way I say." And he blew a strong blast of icy air. The little weathervane shivered with fright and turned wildly all the way around to point in yet another direction. How it wished the north wind would leave.

And then it heard another voice, and this one was soft and sweet but still it had a little chill in it. And this one said, "I am the east wind. When I blow you point that way, and I bring rain, and I bring change and now you will point the way that I blow." And sure enough the little weathervane pointed the way the east wind blew and thought to itself, "Oh, I don't know what to do. I just wait for one wind or another to tell me what to do. In between times, I just twirl around without any direction, and I feel very, very bad about myself. I really don't like myself at all." And so the days passed with the weathervane feeling very sad and still thinking, "Should I be like that one? How will I please this one? Whichever way the wind blows, someone seems to want something different, and I don't know what to do."

As it was sitting there, whirling in one direction and then in another, there came a new voice. And the weathervane said, "Who are you?" This voice said, "Well, I am a part of you. I'm the part of you that's fastened to the top of this barn, and I stay here steady in one place, and I lift up your arms so that you can whirl in one direction or another. And, by the way, I like myself a whole lot." The little weathervane said, "But you just said you're me." And the voice said, "That's right, I'm a part of you, so listen carefully to me. You have a job, and you're doing it well. Your job is to turn with the wind to let people know which way the wind is blowing. But you don't blow with the wind. You stay anchored firmly doing your job. So how come you don't like yourself doing your job so well, letting people know which way the wind is blowing? You should be happy to be you, happy to be such a pretty weathervane, and to be doing your job so well. Please stop fretting about how you ought to be like this one or to be like that one, or ought to decide which way to point or how to behave. Just do what you do so well and so naturally. Point which way the wind is blowing so people will know what to expect of the weather. Let yourself feel strong and flexible doing your job."

The little weathervane listened carefully and after a thoughtful pause said, "I like what you're saying." And the voice replied, "Of course you do. So, now what are you going to do?" And the weathervane said, "Well, I'm going to remember that I am anchored firmly on this barn, and that I do my job very well, and that I don't have to be like a pig or a cow. I don't have to be like a farmer or a milkmaid. I don't have to be like any of the animals here. It is my job to point the way the wind blows, so I think I will just go on doing what I'm doing naturally and happily ever after."

After the story Margo at last began to respond to our work on self-image and self esteem. "The Weathervane" was the beginning of a long series of sessions with me which continued intensively for more than a year. There were many stories told in trance during that time before we began to space the sessions out. As her self-confidence and self-reliance grew she began to make significant changes, starting with progressively longer air flights. Although the flights still evoked feelings of anxiety, these feelings were not prolonged or incapacitating.

She tapered off her sexual encounters outside of marriage, and eventually stopped them entirely. She increasingly participated in activities with her husband and sons. She phased out her dependence on her mother. This last was accomplished slowly and with many traumatic upheavals, which culminated in her mother's angry exit from the household to join her older daughter who lived in another city. At present Margo hopes for a reconciliation on different terms with her mother when enough time has elapsed for a cooler encounter. Margo comes to see me at intervals which are spaced farther and farther apart. At present she is considering a career change. She would like to leave her job (and her boss!). She has been investigating various fields of study offered at the university.

12

The Gardener Who Planted Many Seeds

(A Story for an
Avoidant Personality Disorder)

*H*arold was a "middle child," with an older sister and brother and a younger brother and sister. There were only 13 months in age difference between him and his older brother, and only 12 and a half months in age difference between him and his younger brother. In the first interview Harold described his siblings as being very "smart" and attractive. His older sister, Clarisse, was "the scientist in the family," with an advanced degree in systems engineering and a brilliant career with IBM in research and development. Yes, she was happily married. His older brother, Jim Jr., was "the doctor in the family," a tenured professor in the medical school at Vanderbilt University. He was "the family musician" as well. Yes, he too was happily married and had two children. Harold's younger brother, Tom, was "the lawyer in the family," also forging a distinguished career for himself. Tom was engaged to be married in the spring. His younger sister, Allison, was "the artist in the family" and very gifted.

Harold described himself as the family failure. School work never was easy for him. His teachers were very critical and didn't like him, he said. And Clarisse and Jim Jr. were a "hard act to follow." He was "no good" in sports and always got chosen last to play on a team so he stopped showing up for athletic activities. He was a fat kid in high school and didn't make friends easily. As a matter of fact, he didn't have any friends. None of the girls were interested in him, and he thought they made fun of him among themselves. He had acne. *He wore thick glasses. He was born cross-eyed and had an operation which was only partially successful. He stuttered.*

He was pretty good at math, nothing spectacular, but he decided to go to business school to learn accounting. He now was a bookkeeper in his father's business. He worked alone in a room at the back of the large office. People at work put on a show of being friendly but he "knew" it was because he was the boss's son and wasn't fooled by their overtures. He just kept to himself. Nothing he did was good enough for his father, who rarely spoke to Harold unless he had some criticism to make. His mother was always plaguing him to date her friends' daughters.

As I listened to Harold, I was struck by the contrast between his self-evaluation and his actual appearance. Yes, he did wear thick glasses, but his face was fine-featured and almost handsome. His light brown hair was thick and well-groomed. He was tall, and although he was not muscular, he had a lean, graceful body. I noticed that his hands were long-fingered and almost delicate, but his fingernails were bitten to the quick. He spoke in a barely audible low-pitched voice with an occasional hesitancy rather than a stutter.

The reason he came to see me, he said, was that there was this young woman he met who worked in a nearby office. He was having a lot of trouble with her and was feeling very unhappy. In the ensuing sessions I learned that Diana, the young woman he referred to, began waiting for him after work. One evening she asked him to give her a ride home and when they arrived he accepted her invitation to come in for a drink. After that, she waited for him every evening and she made plans for them, like going to the movies, and once to a jazz concert. Diana was very vivacious and energetic. He found himself looking forward to their evenings. But one of the difficulties was that she was black, and he dreaded his family's

111

reaction. In addition, of late she had stopped arranging to spend every evening with him. It seems she had a very active social life apart from their relationship, and she had begun pursuing her other interests again. He felt rejected and mistrustful. She said, when he asked (which he did repeatedly), that she cared for him but he thought she certainly didn't always act like it. Lately, when he telephoned (he telephoned several times a day), she seemed "la-di-da." When he would stop telephoning, then she would call but he thought it was when she didn't have anything better to do.

At last, Harold told me about his sexual difficulties. He felt unable to initiate a sexual encounter. Unless Diana made the first move, he could not bring himself to make love to her. He became aroused with difficulty and then only when she caressed and stimulated him. He hesitantly confessed that even when he did succeed in having an erection, he often lost it after a short time. Lately, since she started "rejecting" him, he was getting worse. Last weekend they made love Friday night and he performed exceptionally well, but the next morning when Diana wanted to have sex again, he failed. In the afternoon he did pretty well, but that night he failed again. On Sunday morning when he could not manage another erection, Diana got angry and sent him home early, even though they had made plans for the afternoon. He felt lonely and lost.

During these first weeks Harold had been conscientiously listening to the tape we made for him. We had also begun using trance in our sessions. It was at this point that the following story told itself.

O nce upon a time there was a gardener who sat planning his garden late one winter, and he studied a seed catalogue. There he picked out by color and by name whatever struck his fancy among all the beautiful pictures that he saw there. And he chose yellow marigolds and white chrysanthemums. He chose blue larkspur and purple delphiniums. He chose morning glories and asters, and lilies and roses, and many, many others. When he had selected all the many, many different seeds that he wanted to plant, he stood up and with great satisfaction he sent his order off to the big seed store so that he would be ready for the spring planting.

The days passed slowly and he could hardly wait for the seeds to arrive. He was pleased when he felt the weather get warmer and he saw the first robins hopping on the damp earth and pulling the worms. He watched the forsythia pop into yellow bloom overnight, and he saw the first bulbs begin to raise their green shoots above the earth. Everywhere around him were signs that spring was on the way. His impatience grew and grew. At last, in the mailbox one morning, a huge package was delivered. He tore it open with excitement and there spilled out before him dozens of packages of seeds. "Oh," he said, "I can't wait to plant them. I can't wait!" And so he began planting. In rows, and in lovely soft beds, and in back of the house, in front of the house, and around trees, and down in the garden, everywhere, he planted his seeds. As the days passed, he watered and he weeded and he watched and he waited and his heart leapt with happiness whenever he saw another little green shoot push its head above the warm, damp earth. And so the plants grew and grew and he saw, with misgivings, that some grew tall and some did not grow tall. He saw that some bushed out stoutly and some stayed slender, almost skinny. And he watched with doubt as he noticed this one with many leaves and that one with only one or two. He saw this one with long pointed leaves and others with almost circular leaves. And he felt surprise and wonder and also some anxiety about how different the plants were from each other. And he worried that some would not be as beautiful as others, not be as healthy as others, or not be as fine as others.

Each day he leaped up out of bed, impatient to see all the changes that had taken place in the night. And each day he was rewarded with all sorts of new leaves, new growth. Then one day, he began to find buds on many of the plants, and again he felt concern because some buds were fat, and some were little and hard, and some were long and skinny, and some were squat. And he thought, "Oh, my, I wonder if all of them ought to be long and skinny, or maybe they all should be round and squat, or maybe there is something wrong with the ones that are little and shiny and hard." And so he fretted, and he weeded, and he watched, and he waited day by day. When it didn't rain, he watered carefully, and he loosened the earth around the tender stems, and all the time, he wondered and worried secretly that some were so different from others, and he wasn't sure which were doing the thing they ought to be doing. So he watched, and he waited, and he worried, and he worked until one day, he saw a flower. And the next day he saw a hundred flowers. They were all different colors and different shapes, and yes, they were different heights. And he saw that even though they were different, they each were lovely in their own way, and he saw that the round and squat buds became lovely round flowers, and that the long and skinny buds became beautiful slender flutes of flowers, and the little hard shiny ones became little clusters of flowers. And he enjoyed himself because they were all different. He saw that it was all right for them to be different. And so, his heart was full of joy and happiness as each day he saw more and more flowers blooming, bursting with color, and that his garden was especially lovely because there were so many different flowers in it. All the colors seemed to belong together, even though they were so different, one from the other. So he grew very, very proud of his garden. And people came from all over and said, "OH!" and "AH!" and "LOOK!" and "Oh, I like the tall ones best," and others would say, "Oh, but the little ones are sweet and sturdy." And others said, "Well, maybe so, but the ones in the middle, they seem to have all the good things of the tall ones and the good things of the small ones." So everyone picked what they thought were the best, but the gardener smiled because he knew they were all very fine in their own special way.

After the story I learned that, although Harold was employed as a bookkeeper in a deadend job, actually he had an MBA degree. This information was proffered almost apologetically with comments about not ranking very high in his class. Well, actually he was far from being first; he was only in the top ten percentile! His treatment progressed slowly but steadily. He worked very hard at enlarging his range of activities, and through them he gradually developed a circle of acquaintances. He took bridge lessons and joined a bridge club. He became a member of the Audubon Society and joined bird-watching groups. He enrolled in a singles club for professionals. There he met Debbie. Then he ended his relationship with Diana. Eventually I referred him and Debbie to the Masters and Johnson Institute for Sexual Disorders. I reinforced their treatment with hypnotherapy.

Harold, who now asked to be called "Harry," progressed steadily. In less than a year from the time I first saw him, he decided to prepare for the CPA examination. He worked diligently and after months of study he took and passed the difficult exam with a "first" in his own state, and a "ninth" nationally. His father offered him a partnership, which he declined; instead he decided to join a well-established firm of accountants as a junior partner.

It has been several years since we terminated treatment. I hear from Harry from time to time. He and Debbie are married and have a pretty little daughter.

13

The Seedling

(A Story for a Client
Who Had Been Abused as a Child)

Rap did not seek treatment and did not want to come for therapy. He was remanded by the municipal court for wife and child abuse. On probation, he had no choice other than to come for treatment or go to jail.

A skinny, pigeon-breasted man with discolored teeth and a sullen expression, he sat dejectedly and answered in monosyllables. I took it slow and easy. I said that sometimes people mistook me for part of the law enforcement system. I mentioned in passing that I didn't know the judge or the parole officer; I didn't even want to know what the court had to say. I let him know I was interested only in him. He let me know he was not interested. There was nothing I could do for him, in his opinion. He had been "framed." His lousy neighbor who couldn't mind his own damn business had reported him. His neighbor was a liar. His wife was a screamer. Sounded off like she was being murdered if he so much as laid a hand on her. As for his brat kid, he yelled his head off over nothing.

At first Rap played "now you see me, now you don't" with his appointments. His excuses were quite creative. When his parole officer intervened, he would come regularly for a few times. I concentrated on getting his life story and I avoided the subject of the court charges.

When at last he felt safe enough with me, he talked about his childhood. Oldest child of an alcoholic father and an acutely depressed mother, he had to fend for himself at a very early age. His father often flew into a rage and would beat him *brutally with whatever happened to be handy. Once he had fractured Rap's skull with a coal scuttle. Rap felt fiercely protective of his father as far as the outside world was concerned. He never "told on his pa"—not like his own lousy wife and kid.*

When he was a child, his family lived in the country. His father had a job in a factory in town during the week, and worked a large truck garden adjacent to their house on weekends. Rap loved that truck garden. He often thought of owning a farm someday, but guessed that was just another pipe dream like everything else.

It was surprisingly easy for Rap to accept the idea of trance. When he complained about feeling so irritable and nervous that sometimes he felt crazy and out of control, it took only my observation that right now he seemed very tense and nervous for him to agree to "try a way to relax and feel better." When he came out of trance he denied that he had been in trance. He said, "I could hear every word you said; I didn't trance." But after that he would ask for me to "make him feel better," and it was at the very next session that the following story appeared.

O nce upon a time in a faraway place, there stood a very beautiful greenhouse. It was all shining glass and it was enormous. Inside the greenhouse the muted sunlight filtered. The air was wet and warm and everywhere the eye could see, on shelves, hanging from the sides and ceilings, and standing about in big pots on the floor, were beautiful, fragrant, blooming, leafing, living plants of all kinds. There were long rows of flowers of one color and then, next to them, long rows of flowers of another color so that everywhere you looked you saw a profusion of color. And the flowers and the leaves and the plants hung in the delightfully fragrant air. If you stood very still you could hear the muted rustling of growing things and you could reach out your hand to touch the soft petals of one plant, and stroke the shiny sharpness of another, and you could feel the furry stem of another. Everywhere you looked you could see, everywhere you turned you could smell, and hear, and feel the wonder of growing plants all around you.

There was a gardener in charge of this lovely, sunny world. He carefully tended, he carefully watered, he carefully pruned and transplanted and weeded and sorted and cared for the hundreds of plants in this, his enchanted kingdom of the greenhouse. One spring he selected a batch of very choice seedlings and he put each in a little pot of its own, and he put them on a ledge in a special place where he could watch them and tend them in their first delicate days of taking root and establishing themselves as healthy and strong plants. And all went well until one day the little pot at the very end of the row seemed to tip and slip and, without anyone noticing, it had dropped down from the shelf and landed with a soft thud behind a big barricade of pots and plants that completely hid it from view, and there in the semi-darkness it remained, not missed, and not discovered. Its leaves and its stem did not flourish very well because there wasn't much light back there behind the pots and plants that overshadowed it. So it used its strength to grow a huge and vigorous and strong root system. And the root system grew ever stronger and bigger and began to outgrow the confines of the little pot and soon the poor little plant felt choked and cramped and suffocating in the confines of the pot that had grown too small for it. By this time the other plants had long since been taken from their little seedling pots and put into the big, free, warm earth to flourish and to grow strong and big, as was their cycle to do. But our one poor little seedling languished and drooped in the semi-dark, and it seemed as though our poor little plant was doomed.

One morning a fine-looking young boy came into the green-house. He was full of wonder and curiosity as he went down the aisles looking here and there, looking and listening and enjoying the whole colorful, fragrant world. He poked among the leaves and he looked behind the plants, and as he was poking, he noticed a little brown stem peeking out from behind a huge cluster of pots. He exclaimed, "Oh, what have we here? This doesn't look like the rest of the greenhouse. What can this be?" And he reached behind the pots and picked up the little seedling in its tiny cramped pot and brought it out into the light. "Oh," he said, "I think this little plant is lost." And the little plant quivered, struggling for the little boy to hear it whisper, "No, no, I am not lost, not yet, not yet."

And although the little boy didn't hear the words, something in him responded, and he began to turn the little pot this way and that way. Then he noticed that at the very base of the little withered plant there was a small edge of green. "Oh," he said, "let us see. What can be done?" And he took it to the gardener and said, "Look what I have found." "Oh," he said, looking at it, "the poor little thing. It's too late. Let's throw it over here in the trash." "Oh, no," said the young boy. "May I have it?" And the gardener shrugged and said, "If you like, but there are others here I could give you that I think probably would give you more pleasure." He said, "Thank you, but I would enjoy saving this little plant if I can." The gardener replied, "As you wish." And he turned away because he had many important duties.

The young boy carefully broke the pot away from the roots of the little plant. He was amazed to see what big roots it had developed there. And it seemed to him that the root system was very much alive. So he found a place, half-shade and half-sunlight in a bed of rich loam with lots of room, a little apart from the other plants. And he scooped a place for the little plant's roots deep enough to set them firmly in the soil. Gently he separated them and spread them out and then tenderly he dropped fine grains of earth around them until the roots were entirely covered with rich, moist, warm earth and then gently he pressed the earth so that the roots were secure and yet free to grow in all directions.

In the coming days and weeks, that is exactly what they did. They sent out tendrils, they sucked up the moisture, they took nourishment from the earth and sent it up to the light, and soon a sturdy, leafing stem emerged, and the little plant began to grow. The young boy watched it and watered it and tended it carefully, taking delight each day as he saw each new leaf appear until at last the buds began to swell. And with room at last to spread its roots, and with room to spread its stem and leaves, the little plant flowered into the most beautiful plant of all because its root system was so strong.

After the story, Rap became noticeably more responsive, sometimes voluble. Of course, there was much more work for him to do, but the path had been cleared and he was ready to forge ahead. He had alcoholism to deal with as well as paranoia among his multiple deficits and dysfunctions. He joined AA, dropped out, rejoined, fell off the wagon, got on again, and so on. When, after a year's time his parole officer recommended his release from treatment, Rap agreed to come for family therapy with his wife and son. At present I see them at about three-month intervals. I believe that soon we can phase out the sessions altogether.

14

The Island Princess

(A Story for Anorexia Nervosa)

Cynthia came smiling into the room. Tall, thin as a skeleton, with a lovely child-like face and an angelic smile, she stood politely until I asked her to be seated. She told me she came for "help" because her friends with whom she grew up had married, one by one. She felt lonely and left out, anxious because at 29 she had no boy friend. In fact, she had never had a boy friend. She still lived at home with her mother, father, and an older sister. After "finishing school," she had been filling her time with exercise classes, dance classes, jogging, tennis with "the girls," and parties. She also spent a great deal of time with her mother, described as "the dearest person in the world." Her father, an executive vice-president of a world-renowned corporation, was an extremely busy man, rarely at home, often away on business trips. Mother devoted herself to her "volunteer" work, but principally to her daughters, and especially to Cynthia.

In subsequent sessions I learned that Cynthia's sister was obese and behaved "unpleasantly" to her mother, and she was also particularly quarrelsome with Cynthia. She herself had always been an obedient and compliant daughter. Her mother's pet name for her was "Angel." And no boy that Cynthia had brought home could meet mother's high standards for her angel. Mother and daughter had many talks about men, full of dark warnings about men "using" women and then abandoning them. Men, it seemed, had only one goal which they pursued relentlessly. Their main interest, according to mother, was to satisfy their animal sexual needs. A woman must figure out how to keep a man hoping for success in fulfilling his bestial goals without actually allowing him to "go all the way."

Mother admired Cynthia's slenderness and took great pride in her daughter's fashionable appearance. Lately, however, she had felt some alarm because Cynthia had stopped her menstrual cycle. Examination by the family physician elicited a warning that she was far too thin (some 30 pounds under normal weight for her height) and was pushing her dieting and exercising to dangerous levels. Cynthia herself did not consider herself too thin. Actually, she often felt a little fat. And she thought that breasts and hips were "gross."

In subsequent sessions, as she began to come out from behind her social facade, anger toward her sister emerged. When she realized that I accepted her angry feelings without disapproval, other concerns began to surface. Mother, it seems, got drunk every evening on cocktails before dinner. On the rare occasions that her father came home, there were quarrels. Then usually father would slam out of the house. Cynthia would comfort mother and join her with a drink.

We began hypnotherapy mainly focused on body image, developmental cycles, and self-love. She grew more trusting of me and began to become increasingly restless about her life situation. At this point, I told the following story.

T his is a story about a tribe that lived on a beautiful island, once upon a time. And the tribe, although it had many families, lived like one family. And they all felt very closely related to each other. Now in this tribe of families, there was a beautiful, young princess. She was the daughter of the tribal chieftan. Her mother, the first wife of the chieftan, was beautiful, and her chieftan-father was wise and stern. He seemed to be separate from the other people in the tribe. He had his own cares, his own pursuits, and his own work apart from the others. And his wife was often lonely. Sometimes she felt angry because she loved the chieftan and she wished that he would choose to spend more time with her. And so, because she was lonely and because she felt the need for more love, she singled out the young princess to fulfill her happiness. The days passed peacefully except that, from time to time, the young princess felt restless and anxious. Sometimes she would have dreams, and in the dreams she was a young bird, a young bird who would fly away, up, up into the clouds, freely winging into the far horizon. Then the little princess would awaken feeling guilty and anxious again, thinking of her mother, and thinking of the little bird, and disturbed by her restlessness and growing unhappiness.

Whenever the little princess would seek out her playmates, her mother would say, "Be careful, dear. Remember you are a princess. Be careful that harm does not come to you. There are hurtful things in life, and you must be careful of the young men who are not yet warriors, lest they hurt you." But she did not explain in what mysterious way they could hurt her. Then the little princess would ask, "But, mother, they seem pleasant and cheerful. How will they hurt me?" Her mother would frown darkly and say, "They are male, and they could hurt you. You must guard your body from them." The little princess would look at her young body, but she could not understand what she needed to guard. The other young maidens played freely. They wrestled and jostled and threw pebbles at each other. They laughed when they jumped into the ocean. They splashed and they swam and they ducked each other. They had so much fun. But the little princess always stayed close to her mother. And she began to understand that in some mysterious way, her mother seemed to need her. Her mother needed her because she felt sadness in her marriage to the chieftan. Sometimes, when she was alone, the little princess would weep tears. But as she grew into beautiful womanhood, her mother became ever more closely guarding of her, more jealous, more needy of constant companionship.

The other women of the tribe began to notice this. They gathered together and they whispered uneasily that it was time for their young princess to grow into womanhood, but that something seemed to be wrong in the chieftan's hut. As they whispered and they conferred, each began to whisper in her husband's ear for him to notice that the young princess did not play with the other children of the tribe, did not seek a mate, seemed to withdraw more and more. They whispered that the young princess grew thinner and thinner, quieter and quieter, sadder and sadder. Their concern grew until finally the men of the tribe decided to seek a conference with the chieftan. They told him their fears about what they observed, but he replied gruffly, "Nonsense, nonsense, I am the chief. My princess is fine. I will not have anything wrong with her! My wife is fine, too, and you will hold your criticism. Mind your own business." They all withdrew, shaking their heads sadly. That night they told their wives that the chieftan was not to be disturbed.

And so the days followed one after the other, and it became time for the princess to choose a mate, but she had not learned to know any young man. She was afraid of all the young men, and she had come to understand that her mother had been warning her about having loving sex with men, so that now her body shrank in fear from the idea. And she was so afraid, so very afraid that she even stopped her monthly cycle so that she could stay a little princess by her mother's side, and never grow up to join the other young women, never grow up to someday be, herself, the queen of the tribe.

This sad state of affairs had gone on for many moons, when one day a strange and beautiful canoe approached the island. In the canoe sat a very, very old, old man. They recognized, by markings on his face and chest and by his elaborate headdress, that he was a very great chieftan indeed. His canoe was paddled by three stalwart young warriors, beautiful of body and intelligent of mind. The villagers gathered, and the whole tribe murmured and waved and wondered aloud as the canoe drew nearer. As it approached the shore, the foremost young warrior stood up, muscular and handsome, and with his paddle made the sign of peace in the air. A great shout went up from the tribe on shore and they began their lyrical song of welcome. As the music swelled over the waves, the canoe came gently to rest on the shore, and the young warriors leapt out into the shallow waters and pulled it up onto the sand. Then, courteously and respectfully they lifted the old chieftan out upon the dry and golden shore. He stood there, dignified, slowly shifting his intense gaze from face to smiling face.

Then the chieftan of the island tribe came forward and the two men made between them the gracious formal sign between chieftans. Only then did the chieftan of the island tribe speak. "You have come and honored us with your presence. Pray, tell us what mission you serve and how we can serve you, honored chieftan." And the great chieftan replied, "There has spread among the islands the story of a beautiful young princess here on your island who is now growing into womanhood. I have brought three of my stalwart warrior sons so that they may meet, and she may choose. We hope that we will have a joining of the tribes, for we have no young princesses on our island for them."

The island chieftan said, "Yes, indeed, I have a daughter." And he turned to his wife asking her to bring the princess forward. But the princess hung back. She tried to hide behind her mother. Her mother came slowly, reluctantly, to stand by the chieftan's side, for she was afraid to disobey him. But tears stood in her eyes and she held tightly to her daughter's hand. The little princess began to weep bitterly. The ancient chieftan looked at her, and his sons looked at each other in dismay. Then the ancient chieftan said, "She is very beautiful, but I expected a young woman, and this is a small child." The island chieftan said, "No, honored chieftan, this is a young woman who is old enough and ready for wedlock." The chieftan's wife whispered, "No, no."

And the little princess shook her head miserably, as she slowly lowered it. But as she did, she peeked out of the corner of her eye at the three young warriors, and the youngest seemed very fair to her indeed. As she continued to steal glances at him, she saw that his body was strong and beautiful, his face handsome and intelligent, and his eyes were deep as the dark waters of the sea. She saw that his hands were sensitive, and his feet were well-shaped and slender. So, taking courage, she shyly came out from behind her mother and stood taller. She raised her eyelids and looked straight into his eyes. Then he smiled, and in spite of her fear, she could not stop her lips from smiling back.

The wise old chieftan saw this, and he said to the island chief, "I think perhaps she is soon to be a woman." The island chieftan replied, "Indeed she is. And I hope she finds favor in your eyes." The wise old chieftan said, "I will make a test for her. If she will take her own canoe and paddle alone out into the beautiful waters to a nearby island, and if there she will make her way, unknown as a princess, among the peoples who dwell there, and if there she will make maiden friends, and if there she will make warrior friends, and if there she will bloom into womanhood, if one year from today she will have found her own way, apart from the protection of her mother and her tribe, then one year from today we shall return and pledge our troth."

The chieftan looked at his daughter and she looked up at him. He could see that, although she was afraid, still she hoped for his consent. She dared not look at her mother because she could feel her mother's body trembling. So she looked again at the young warrior. Her heart leaped up, and for the first time, she let go of her mother's hand. Then something wonderful took place. She saw the chieftan reach for her mother's hand and hold it. Her heart felt light and free as the bird of her dreams. She felt impatient to begin her adventures.

It was time for the chieftan and his sons to depart. The islanders began the dancing and singing of "Farewell, farewell, return to us soon." The chieftans performed the ceremony of parting, and as the sun began to set at the golden rim of the ocean, the ancient chieftan and his stalwart sons glided out into the shimmering water on their homeward journey.

The next weeks were spent preparing the young princess for her voyage. She felt afraid, especially at night when she retired to her little hut alone. But the excitement of painting designs on her canoe, and on her paddle, of selecting garments for her journey, all the many preparations gave her courage.

At last the day came for her departure. The singing people of her island cheered and waved as she paddled away from them, alone in her newly decorated canoe, sitting alone among the garlands of flowers that filled the canoe.

Cynthia came out of trance relaxed and smiling. She wanted to know what happened to the princess after the story. I said, "There is a sequel which will follow, in time." In the next few sessions, we talked about possible careers she might pursue. The idea of studying to become a professional fashion model appealed to her. She also arranged to attend a ballet class which met at cocktail time, and so appeared for dinner at home only after the drinking hour. Next, she telephoned two friends she had not seen for some time. She went to a party, something she had begun to avoid. She met a young man she liked, and although she felt frightened, she did not bring him home to meet mother.

And then, the sequel to the first story told itself.

This is the second part of the story of the Island Princess. You remember she paddled alone in her lovely painted canoe, heaped with flowers, cheered on by the singing people of her island. And she looked back to wave goodbye once more to her anxious mother and her smiling chieftan father. She went out full of fear, and yet eager for the adventures that her new voyage would bring her. She understood that it was the voyage into her womanhood, and when she returned, after her experiences, that the handsome young warrior prince who had met her gaze and set her heart to pounding, would be waiting there to ask her hand in marriage. And she began seeing herself in her mind's eye, lovely in her bridal dress, with wreaths of flowers about her neck and a symbolic orchid in her hair, seeing herself on her wedding day, standing beside her handsome young warrior prince. And with this beautiful picture in her mind, she paddled harder and stronger toward the far island where she would learn the ways of being a woman. It was hard to separate from her mother and her father, and she was afraid, but she knew that if she would learn the ways of women, she must go to another place among young women of another island where she would no longer be seen as a little child, but be accepted as what she really is, a young and blooming woman.

After many, many, many hours of paddling, when she began to feel very, very tired, there in the distance she saw the mountains and the palm trees of an island rising from the waters of the sea. This gave her new energy, and she paddled harder. Soon she could make out figures of men and women on the shore. They had sighted her and were waiting, forming a circle with arms intertwined, awaiting her arrival. When at last her canoe was within hailing distance, young men of the island ran through the water, waded out shoulder height, took hold of the sides of her canoe and drew her gently ashore. She stood in the canoe and looked about her. She saw a shining island filled with flowers, trees in leaf, singing birds, and as she looked from face to face of the waiting islanders, she saw that there were many young women just like her, and she stood smiling into the eyes and faces of her new friends. They drew her into their circle, and her heart grew lighter as she felt the warmth of their welcome. Her curiosity and eagerness to learn her new ways welled up inside her.

And so her days began on the island. There she learned the gentle but self-sufficient ways of being a woman. She took charge of her own food gathering and preparation, and she learned from the others how to cook many delectable dishes. She learned how to hunt and to gather food. She learned how

to sew sails for the canoes. She even learned how to plait
banana leaves to make shelter. She learned to tend the fire,
she learned to make pots to cook in, she learned to weave
cloth, and oh, what fun to learn to draw the beautiful designs
and then to make the handsome rich dyes with which to
decorate the cloth she wove for her garments.

And each day she grew stronger and more confident as her
skills grew in the womanly arts. The young men in the village
understood that she was there as if in a school, and so they
were kind, and they joked and they played, and she had many
friendly encounters, lovely sings in the moonlight, and wonderful lazy hours swimming in the lagoon. Sometimes she
would put her face down in the water and when she opened
her eyes there were many colored fish swimming below her.
She would raise her head from the water and laugh out loud
with delight thinking how she would make designs like that
for the cloth that she wove.

Her days passed cheerfully and happily and each day she
grew more and more skillful. She learned that the seasons had
a cycle. There was a time for planting and a time for growing
and a time for harvesting, a time for work, and a time for play.
The sun had a cycle, and the moon had a cycle, and the waves
came in and rolled back in an orderly rhythm, and the tide
had a cycle for high tide and low tide. And she found that she
too had a cycle, a womanly cycle of fertility and fruition, and
she began with pride and with pleasure her monthly cycle
which heralded her womanhood. When her monthly cycle
first began, the whole village celebrated. They made a sacrifice
to the gods of fertility, thanking the gods for the young princess' well-being and her maturation into womanhood. And she
herself felt very proud. There were stars in her eyes. And that
evening she sat quietly by the dying fire, dreaming dreams
of her young prince, her husband-to-be.

One day her new friends formed a circle about the grass hut in which she sat thinking about her young prince. They began to sing a song which she recognized as their loving song of "Farewell, farewell, until we meet again." She sprang to her feet in surprise and then her heart swelled inside her chest with excitement as she understood that they were telling her that she had finished her task. Her journey into womanhood was completed and soon it would be time to return home to her island to begin the next part of her life.

With fast-beating heart she dressed in her finest woven dress with the most beautiful fish designs. The colors glowed, but not more so than her lovely face, not more so than the aura of energy and love that surrounded her from head to foot. The islanders pulled her canoe to the water's edge, and she saw with delight that they had newly painted the designs, and now among the old symbols and patterns on her canoe were added the new designs of the island and her womanhood. She stepped proudly into her canoe, and accepted from them the wreaths of flowers, and their gifts. She carefully lowered, into the bow, the pots she had made, and looked with pride at all the symbols of her skills and her maturity.

When at last she began to paddle slowly away, it was the sound of the voices of her new friends bidding her, "fare-thee-well, fare-thee-well, go, go with our love, sweet princess," and so she paddled faster then, making a straight line directly into the golden path cast across the sea by the radiant sun. She paddled with her new strength, and she could feel the energy in her womanly body. The return journey was easier than it had been when first she started out. And after long hours which she spent in dreaming visions of her new life as a woman, and almost before she expected it, she recognized the familiar peaks and ravines of her own home island rising gradually from the sea before her eyes. Straining her gaze and shading her eyes with her hands, she could make out the tall, long body of her chieftan father, and beside him the soft shape of her mother, and soon she drew close enough to make out the faces of all her tribe, and then, one by one, to make out all the familiar landmarks of her childhood.

And so she paddled faster and stronger, her heart racing with joy and excitement, eager to show her tribe how she had grown into womanhood. When at last they drew her canoe onto the golden sand, she stepped out strong and erect and ran to greet her mother and father. As she stood before them and made the sign of respect and love, first to one and then the other, she stepped back and looked into her father's eyes and then into her mother's eyes. There she read their pride and their joy in her. And then she noticed that her mother still clasped the hand of her father. And she felt the warmth of her joy that they welcomed her back with pride.

She dared not ask after the young prince warrior, and smiling, she waited until all the songs of greeting had been sung. Then the villagers parted, making a path for her between their ranks. At the edge of the village she saw revealed a most splendid dwelling. It was hung with the most elaborate banners and wreaths of flowers. The handsomest of woven mats covered the threshold. And as she looked upon this festive shelter, to her surprise and her amazement she saw standing before it the ancient chieftan who had offered his warrior son in marriage if she should prove herself no longer a child but grown to full womanhood. She drew herself to her full height. She was indeed beautiful, tall and slender, brilliantly garbed in the cloth of her own design, womanly, womanly from the crown of her head to the soles of her delicate feet.

The ancient chieftan came forward slowly, stopped, and made the formal sign of greeting and respect. She knelt before him and responded with the sign, in return, of greeting and respect. Then he bade her rise to her feet, and slowly turning, summoned the young prince warrior who stepped from the shadows of the banners and stood hesitantly for one moment on the threshold of the beautiful shelter. When his eyes beheld the womanly form and beautiful face of the young princess, he glowed with love and admiration. As he drew himself to his fullest manly height, his father bade him advance, greet the young princess and pay his respect. When the prince and princess had greeted each other formally, the whole island burst into song. It was the nuptial song of love and commitment. The two chieftans stood facing each other as they pledged their honor to each other. Henceforth, their clans would be joined and their tribes be friends in war and peace, when their two finest, the prince and the princess, were joined in wedlock.

And then the marriage ceremony began. All the islanders wreathed themselves in flowers. Fragrant woods were burned in great bonfires on the beach, wreaths were woven, mats were laid. And the villagers began their ceremonial dances, clapping and singing, circling slowly about the young pair at first, and then gradually quickening their pace until the dance spun faster and faster, more and more exhilarated. Their singing rose higher and higher and the clapping, and the leaping, and the dancing grew wilder and freer, until at last, in the small hours of the morning, when the celebration had subsided, the ancient chieftan took the hand of his son and joined it to the hand of the princess. They pledged their troth of holy marriage. Then the whole island tribe began feasting, and toasting, dancing and singing, and the celebration went on for seven days and seven nights. On the seventh night, the young prince gathered his young bride in his arms and carried her to his canoe. There stood the ancient chieftan with her father and mother. They embraced her and the young prince and bade them farewell in their new life, until they should meet again. Happily paddling away, to the rhythm of songs drifting lazily across the water, they paddled their canoe together to their new island where they lived happily ever after.

Cynthia continued to come to see me for more than a year. As she began to make changes, her mother became increasingly opposed to her continuing treatment with me. She complained, both to me and to Cynthia, that she could see no progress and thought Cynthia was simply wasting money. Invited to come to sessions with Cynthia, she came only twice, both times with reluctance and hostility. One of her comments, which she made several different times, was, "That sounds like something straight out of a book." To which I twice replied, "Quite right. I often learn from books."

Cynthia enrolled in a fashion modeling school. Soon she was modeling for a fashion photographer. She continued treatment, and within six months she was earning enough to move into an apartment with another young woman whom she met at school. When she terminated treatment, she had gained 20 pounds, had restored her menstrual cycle, and was happily dating a young man.

15

The Roman Princess

(A Story for a Bulimic)

Miriam was pretty, "pleasingly plump," doe-eyed, and gentle of speech. She told a tale of distress and shame. Her father was a prominent brain surgeon whose professional life left him little time for his wife and two daughters. Her mother devoted her time to her daughters and the social life befitting the wife of such an eminent husband. Fashionable clothes and, above all, a fashionable body, suitably slender, were an important part of daily life. Stringent dieting was routine in that household. Propriety and conformity were the cardinal virtues, with the tacit goal of arranging "appropriate" marriages for the two daughters. It was understood that they would protect themselves from the evil designs of lecherous men and would "save themselves" for their husbands.

In her early teens, Miriam began secretly bingeing. She covertly consumed enormous quantities of food, mostly "junk" food, fast food, cookies, doughnuts, candy and whatever she could raid from the refrigerator and pantry. She spent her entire allowance on food as well. After her daily gorging, usually late at night, she would retire to the bathroom, put a finger down her throat, and vomit it all up. She felt guilty and filled with shame over her "disgusting" behavior. She lived in terror of being caught. She became an accomplished liar.

Then she met a young man and entered into a sexual relationship with him. She knew her parents would find him unsuitable. In addition to his general unacceptability, he was also an alcoholic. He became intoxicated regularly and often embarrassed her in public. *Although she wanted to terminate the relationship, she could not seem to summon enough resolve to give up the emotional support he afforded her in his sober moments. She desperately wanted "help" with her "shameful compulsion," and my support in separating herself from her lover.*

She proved to be very responsive to trance induction, and we succeeded in establishing a trusting rapport after a relatively short period of time, during which we did not approach the issues of bulimia or sex. Treatment was centered around acceptance of her body and permission to acknowledge her own feelings and thoughts as valid. She continued her stormy relationship, and she continued bingeing and vomiting. Then, at last, in the twelfth session, the following story appeared.

This is a story about the daughter of a noble Roman Senator, a young princess born into a noble household. Her mother was a lady — high-born and of important station, of prominent social position in Roman society at a time when Rome ruled the world, all the civilized world, and was reaching out to rule the barbarians as well. What was so very remarkable about this society was that they made their own laws and the laws of their society were made in order to please themselves. So they felt very virtuous, very virtuous indeed, and since the goal of life in their society was pleasure, those Romans who knew how to pursue pleasure in living were regarded as highly virtuous and were most admired, while those who did not know how to pursue pleasure and who were sad and serious were looked down upon and were ostracized.

To go back to our story, the little princess grew up in her parents' noble household . . . a very, very beautiful household with marble halls, with inlaid mosaic floors, with many slaves. Her life was delightful, ordered, and full of joy. And eagerly, day by day, she would observe the ways of her elders. They would go to the games and there they would applaud stalwart, brave gladiators who fought the wild and ferocious beasts. The nobility would clap and laugh and reward their acts of valor. And when the circus was done, they would come back to their sumptuous palaces and begin their feasting. Roman banquets would last far into the night, with course after course of food, goblet after goblet of wine, and they all ate and drank enormously. They laughed, and they joked, and they enjoyed themselves very much.

Then, when their stomachs felt uncomfortably full or they felt uncomfortably intoxicated, they would repair to very special rooms — the ladies to one, the gentlemen to another. These were very large and very elegant rooms, and they were known as the vomitoria. The ladies would retire into their own beautiful room that had elaborate mosaics lining the walls; soft music played, slaves stood ready with perfumed cloths and basins. There the ladies would daintily put their fingers down their throats and would delicately and gracefully vomit into the basins which the slaves would then remove. Other basins with perfumed water and floating flower petals were instantly offered, and the ladies gently wiped their faces and their mouths. Whereupon flacons of water laced with lemon rounds were ready, and they would rinse their mouths, delicately gargle, and spit into the basin, which the slaves then deftly removed. Finally, the ladies would seat themselves before the long mirrors, and the slaves would comb and brush their hair into elaborate curls, and powder and rouge their pretty faces. The ladies had learned to vomit so precisely that they never, never splattered or stained their fine embroidered dresses.

144

And when they had completed the entire elaborate function, they would repair back to the tables where the gentlemen, who had just been completing the same ritual, would greet them. Feeling delightfully light and empty, they would start their feasting all over again. And they would continue through the night. The young princess watched and longed for the day when she, too, could join the society of grownups and enjoy the pleasures of the games and feasting. She knew that she would have to learn the art of vomiting gracefully and delicately, but she assumed that her mother would teach her in time.

And it came to pass that one day the lovely young princess experienced her first menstrual cycle. She was delighted and ran to report to her mother. Her mother giggled and hugged her and said, "My goodness, my goodness, now you're beginning to be a woman. What fun!" And the little princess laughed, and was also joyous, and she said, "And now, mother, will you teach me all the arts of being a woman?" And her mother said, "Well of course, my dear. What fun!" And so the little princess began her studies. Her mother taught her graces of conversation, the graces of table manners, and above all, the grace of knowing when she had had enough at the table, not too much but just enough, so that then she would go and relieve herself. Her mother would teach her, in private, the art of vomiting gracefully and neatly so as not to appear gross or indelicate, and above all, not to soil or spot her clothes or offend anyone with her vomiting.

And the young princess was a wonderful pupil. She learned her lessons quickly and well, and she repeatedly asked her mother, "Now, mother, am I ready to join the grownups? Now am I ready?" So that at last, on her sixteenth birthday, her mother smiled on her and said, "I will speak to your father, and if he approves, tonight you shall join us at the banquet table." And so the noble lady conferred with her husband, who, when he heard her request, smiled with surprise and said, "So soon? But of course."

So the mother and the young princess together chose a charming gown and together prepared her for her first banquet. That night she joined the grownups at the banquet table. She watched covertly what everyone did, and she observed that everyone was full of laughter and pleasure and that everyone was enjoying himself. Oh, she was very pleased to be there! She continued to watch carefully and take heed of the time when she would cease to feel pleasure in eating, in drinking, and be aware that it was time to go to the vomitorium. And sure enough, as soon as she felt uncomfortably full, she glanced at her mother. Her mother nodded, and she excused herself politely, and went, for the first time, to the special room.

The slaves smiled at each other and winked when she came in, and giggled because she had at last joined the grownups. They held a basin for her and, although she felt a little uneasy, she knew her mother had taught her well, and so, gracefully, she put her two fingers down her throat, and skillfully, easily, without a single splash, she vomited neatly into the basin. The slaves looked at each other with approval of what a fine lady with great manners she had become. They whisked the basin away, and brought her a goblet of lemon and water. She rinsed her mouth ever so daintily and gargled in ever so ladylike a manner and spat into the basin which the slaves again whisked away. And then two slaves handed her perfumed warm cloths to wipe her lips and face, and when they took them from her, she seated herself on a low curved bench before the tall mirrors. Two slaves rearranged her hair, rearranged her makeup, smoothed her gown, and bowed as they backed away from her and stood smiling shyly as she thanked them graciously and then went back to the banquet table.

When she was seated again, she noticed directly across the table from her a very handsome young nobleman. He was watching her and so she smiled at him. And he smiled back. But then she noticed that he seemed to be drinking more wine than the others, and he did not go to the vomitorium. She was puzzled by this and then she felt dismayed, because she noticed he was no longer smiling and having fun, but that he seemed cross. He began to quarrel with his neighbors, and she felt sad and disappointed because she had found the young nobleman attractive until he began to behave in so boorish a fashion. She discussed this episode later with her mother, and her mother said she would speak of this to her husband, the Senator.

When her mother mentioned to the Senator that the young princess had looked with favor on the young nobleman but that his boorish behavior had dismayed her, she asked the Senator if he would speak to the young man. And the Senator agreed to do so. And so the following day, he summoned the young nobleman to lunch. Graciously he began talking about life and custom. Then he spoke of his daughter, and how she had looked with favor upon the young nobleman. The young man flushed with pleasure, and then with shining eyes, asked permission to court the beautiful young woman. The Senator did not reply to his request. Instead, he brought the subject around to moderation and to knowing when you have had enough, and to knowing when it is time to get rid of excesses in order to start over again and so to always be able to experience pleasure and enjoyment.

The young man listened attentively, and said, "Noble sire, I don't know how to do that. I have never been taught to do that." The Senator then replied, "There is a secret place in the city. The young noblemen who go there go anonymously so that there will not be any social blame placed on them, and there, together, they learn the art of continence, the art of knowing how much gives pleasure and where pleasure stops. And when you have gone there for a year, come back and perhaps we will consider your petition for the hand of my lovely princess." The young man's eyes lit up again for he had indeed found the princess very desirable.

And so it came to pass that the young man went to the secret place in Rome to learn the art of continence, the art of knowing when to stop because the pleasure stops at that point, and when to make sure that he could continue to experience pleasure in his life. In a year he had learned his lesson well and came back to report to the Senator. The Senator was very pleased with the young nobleman and called his wife and the young princess to meet with him. When the princess came into the room her heart fluttered. She felt great pleasure. Her mother smiled with happiness too. And then, in the presence of her two parents, the young princess and the handsome young nobleman, who both had learned the art of continence, pledged their troth. In Roman society they called it the art of experiencing pleasure; in other societies, they call it happiness. Whether it is known as pleasure or as happiness, it comes from the approval of our peers and the way we feel about ourselves, and so, these two young people had learned the secret of happiness, or, as they called it, pleasure. And they lived pleasurably (happily) ever after.

Among other messages, this paradoxical story gave permission and took the shame out of bingeing and vomiting. Bulimia could no longer serve as a rebellion against the strictures of her mother's standards. After this story session, Miriam began one by one to report the following changes. First of all, she decided that she would leave the house whenever she felt the urge to binge because she realized that she binged only when she was alone, never in public. Soon she reported that she binged and vomited only three or four times a week. She joined a health club and began to exercise regularly. To her delight, not only did she not gain weight but, on the contrary, she began to slim down. She joined Al-Anon and learned new ways to deal with alcoholics. She finally ended her relationship with her alcoholic lover when he refused to go to Alcoholics Anonymous meetings. Later, he did join AA and became a recovering alcoholic, but Miriam had lost interest in a love relationship with him. Over the months, she made new friends and found new, interesting activities. For example, she joined an amateur theatrical group and became involved with a community theater. Finally, she got a job and moved out of her parental home. After little more than a year, she had stopped all bingeing and vomiting.

I have used variations of this story with other bulimic clients, always adjusting it, of course, to the special needs of each individual.

16

Journey From a Frozen Land

(A Story for an Obese Client)

Annabelle began sobbing almost as soon as she sat down. Between sobs and shudders she told me about her feelings of despair because her mother constantly criticized her, quarreled, cursed, and scolded her. As she talked, sobbed, and gradually calmed herself, I closed my eyes and heard an angry little girl about 13 years old. In fact, Annabelle stood almost six feet tall, weighed at least 300 pounds, and was somewhere in her mid-thirties. Yes, she lived with her mother; yes, she worked at a monotonous job for minimum wages; no, she had no friends. Sobs again. Her efforts to lose weight had all ended in failure. Two years ago she had a gastroplasty operation, a procedure in which the stomach is stapled together to make it very small. After the operation she lost 80 pounds, but within a year's time she began to gain them back again, and she now had gained over 100 pounds. Her surgeon suggested that she undergo a second operation, but before she subjected herself to that, she decided to come to see me.

Our sessions were scheduled on a once-a-week basis, and for some 20 weeks were targeted on assertiveness and self-esteem. She proved to be responsive and intelligent. It was at this point that the following story appeared.

T his is a story about a young woman who lived in a cold bleak land. In that land, it was always winter. The trees were bare and stood like icy, black sticks in the landscape. The land was barren and frozen, and she lived in a house, by herself. It was very hard to keep warm, so what did she do? She put on layer after layer to bundle herself up, trying to keep warm, so that finally she looked like a large, shapeless ball almost as wide as she was tall, trying to keep warm by adding layer, on layer, on layer. But she was not very happy because she spent all her time trying to keep warm. There was little time or energy for anything else. And still she felt cold and very lonely and very sad.

One day there came a brisk knock on the door. She waddled over slowly and clumsily to open the door, just a crack, so as not to let in too much cold, and as she peeked out fearfully, she asked, "Who is there?" A strong and firm voice replied, "What are you doing here? Did you not get our notice that everyone is being evacuated from this place? Come with me immediately." But the young woman said to the man, "Oh, no, I can't leave my house. I'm afraid to leave the house." The strong voice insisted, "Nonsense, you must leave or you will perish here." And the stranger forced the young woman to come with him. Fearfully she waddled out, and they started on a journey. After a while, she asked, "Where are you going? What will I do?" And the voice answered, "Trust in me. I am taking you to a land where you can be warm and happy." But the young woman, who had never known warmth or happiness, felt very fearful, and yet, she understood that she had no choice so she waddled on as fast as she could after the stranger. They were following a path that led through all the desolation and they proceeded in this way for many days.

One morning, the young woman noticed that the landscape seemed to be changing. Here and there, she saw shrubs, and some of them had leaves — she had never seen such a sight before! She noticed also that she had moisture on her forehead and in the palms of her hands, and moisture trickled down her body from her armpits. And so she asked the stranger, "What is this moisture on my forehead and on my hands, and trickling down my body?" The stranger laughed, "Ha, ha," with amusement. "You are sweating, my dear." "Oh," said the young woman, "what is sweating?" And the stranger said, "When your body gets warm, in order to cool it off, it sends out moisture which is called sweat, and when the moisture evaporates, you get cooler." "Oh," said the young woman with wonder, "am I too warm?" And the stranger said, "Try taking off a layer or two and see how you feel."

So timidly, with many fears, the young woman took off the top two layers, and oh, she felt much more comfortable and much lighter immediately. She also found that she felt freer, and then she found that she could walk better and enjoy the landscape more. Each day, with wonder and with growing delight, she saw many new things appear as they proceeded on their journey — leaves on the trees, little animals hopping about. The sun appeared, golden and radiant, and the sky was blue — nothing like anything she had ever noticed before. And she said to the stranger, "We are in a new country." The stranger smiled and replied, "Yes, the climate is changing, and I notice that you have more sweat on your brow."

And so the young woman, this time with much less fear and with some eagerness, took off another two layers. Oh, and she felt wonderful! Much lighter. She was able to walk much better, and the stranger did not have to stop and wait for her nearly so often. She could swing her arms freely, and her legs felt longer, and she noticed each day that there were more trees in leaf, more flowers in bloom, more birds winging, more song. The breeze was fragrant and delightful on her face, and without waiting for the stranger to suggest it, she began taking off layer after layer, and freeing her body more and more.

One day, they arrived in a land of beautiful gardens in full bloom. Everywhere she looked there were gardens surrounding her. And when she looked down, she saw herself, her own true self, her slender self, emerging from all the layers, and she saw that she was beautiful. She saw and felt her beauty and her freedom. She felt exhilarated with energy. She wanted to dance and sing. The stranger seemed to read her mind and said, "Yes, do dance and sing, my dear. Do feel your wonderful energy, your glow of happiness, your delight in your slenderness." And so the young woman began to skip and whirl and leap and run. Sometimes she would run ahead of the stranger and then she would stop to look back laughing, and sometimes she would dance circles around the stranger, feeling full of glee and mischief, and sometimes she would run back to pick a flower and put it in her shining hair. Sometimes, smiling and laughing, she would gather flowers and present them to the stranger. She felt so happy to be free that she said to the stranger, "Let us stop here. This is so lovely." And the stranger said, "Not yet, my dear. We are almost there, but not quite." The young woman asked, with wonder in her eyes, "What other delights could there be?" The stranger smiled wisely and said, "You will see, my dear, you will see."

One morning, they came into a city of shining buildings and luxuriant gardens. And there all about her everywhere, the young woman saw others, slender and beautiful like her. They greeted her, and they welcomed her, and they asked for her name. Timidly she asked their names in return. And they invited her to join in their dances and their singing, and they included her in their family, and that is how she became part of the wonderful community that dwells among the gardens. She learned to share and to work with them. She learned to play and sing with them. Then one day, she singled out a particular person, who also seemed to single her out. They joined hands and decided to be special to each other. And so the young woman lived happily ever after.

After the story, Annabelle began to make noticeable changes. She joined the YWCA and swam three times a week. She began programming a balanced, low-calorie diet, which we reinforced each session with hypnotherapy. To date she has taken off 110 pounds. She began to show interest in her clothes. She bought colored contact lenses which made her irises appear a lovely deep green. She enrolled in a night class at a junior college. She learned to practice autohypnosis, with which she reinforced our sessions. She began to make friends, first in her job, and then at school. She started to job hunt.

When I last heard from Annabelle she telephoned to invite me to her wedding! I most certainly will be there.

17

The Boy Who Lost His Way

(A Story for
Substance Abuse: Alcoholism)

*R*ick *called for an appointment but failed to appear for it. Two weeks later he called again, explaining that he had lost his nerve, but now was feeling so miserable that he hoped I would be willing to give him another chance.*

He appeared a half an hour too early, and was waiting in the reception room when I first saw him, a man about 40 years old. His suit was ill-fitting, and his shirt had a frayed collar. His shoes were worn and unpolished. His fingernails were dirty. He was smoking a cigarette nervously, disregarding the "Thank You For Not Smoking" sign on the wall opposite him.

When he sat down in my office, I asked him to put out his cigarette. He frowned and protested that he could not "get himself together" if he couldn't smoke. I explained that when we smoke, we "blow away our feelings," and that he had come to a place where being in touch with our feelings is impor-tant. I added that if he wished he could interrupt our session and go out into the corridor to smoke, but of course he would be using his time for smoking instead of working with me. He said, "Okay," but he did not leave during the session.

He told a hard-luck story of lost jobs, unreasonable bosses, a hostile wife who got a divorce and kept his children from seeing him. His brother and two sisters refused to help him anymore. Even his parents seemed to be turning against him. The whole world was against him! He was out of money with no place to stay, now that even friends closed their doors to him.

I asked what he thought had made all this happen. He said, "I never did have any luck." I asked if he could recall when his luck first began to run out. After some prodding on my part, he told the story of a wild, rebellious adolescence, parents who gave him material support but no love, an impulsive early marriage, and jobs from which he got fired for "no reason." And at last, naturally, when he really felt low, he would drink to feel better, just like everybody else. Now his only consolation was to drink. Yes, he drank every day. His parents told him that unless he saw a "shrink" they would wash their hands of him, "So, here I am."

I asked if he had ever attended an Alcoholics Anonymous meeting. He said his ex-wife and his parents went to Alanon but he would not go to AA himself. Just a lot of drunken bums went there. And besides, he didn't go for this religious stuff.

I said that if he wanted to start treatment with me he would have to attend at least two AA meetings a week. He protested that he was not an alcoholic. He could stop whenever he wanted. He just didn't want to right now. Drink was the only comfort he had. I waited. He asked if I would see him without AA meetings if he stopped drinking. I said, no, because my experience with patients who drink too much and refused to join AA was completely negative, and so I was unwilling to waste my time or his. I explained that stopping a drinking habit without an experienced support group was too difficult. I suggested that he think it over and let me know what he decided to do. Almost immediately he said, okay, he had decided and when should he come back for his next appointment. I gave him an appointment with the stipulation that he attend two AA meetings before he was due to return, or I would not see him.

He did not show up, nor did I hear from him for almost three months. When finally he called, he said, "I have joined

AA and now will you let me come to see you?" When he came in, he looked frail, gaunt and sick. He had lost a great deal of weight. He told me that the month before he had suffered an attack of delirium tremens which so terrified him that he entered the detoxification ward of a hospital where he stayed for almost three weeks. When he left the hospital he joined AA and now, at last, was ready to admit to being an alcoholic and needing help.

The following sessions were involved with establishing trust, providing supportive encouragement, and the beginning of goal-setting.

He joined an AA bowling team. He got a job delivering newspapers. He began recovering his physical strength. We started hypnotherapy. Metaphoric use of the AA Twelve Steps supplied rich material for trance and change.

Then he "fell off the wagon." He missed two appointments. When at last he called, he said he had bumped into a couple of old friends and had a few beers. He lost his job. But he was back at AA again, and could he come in to see me?

When he arrived for his session, the following story presented itself.

O nce upon a time, there was a very small boy who lost his way in the deep forest. And the more he tried to find his way back out again, the deeper he went into the forest and the more lost he became. Although he didn't realize it, he was going around and around in circles. And he was very frightened. The tears were coursing down his face as he grew very tired,

and he began to sob more and more deeply and slowly. All
at once, he saw a little clearing, and in the middle of it, a small
hut. His spirits lifted as he ran to the hut and knocked on the
door. A deep voice answered, "Come in. It's open. It's always
open."

So the little boy pushed the door open and peered into the
dim room. As his eyes grew accustomed to the half-light, he
saw sitting at the table in the corner a very large and very old
man. The old man thumped on the table and said, "Well, come
in, come in. What are you waiting for? Come in. All are welcome here." And so the little boy went in and stood a few
paces away from the old man, who asked, "Are you lost, little
boy?" The little boy nodded his head miserably. Then the old
man said, "Well, well, you're safe here. Sit down, sit down. I
have a magic potion." The little boy looked up with wonder.
And the old man said, "Well, here, I'll pour you some." He
poured a liquid into a small glass, and the little boy drank it.
In a few moments he felt exhilarated. He felt as though he
were in a large and beautiful room, and as though he were
eight feet tall. His spirits lifted, and he felt cheerful, powerful, and very, very safe.

But in a few moments he seemed to doze, and then to sleep,
and when he awakened, he felt sick. He had a terrible head-
ache, and he felt queasy in his stomach. The old man looked
at him with twinkling eyes and chuckled, "Ho, ha, ha," and
said, "you need another magic potion. Drink it down." And
the little boy, feeling so sick, reached for it and drank it down.
And it was, indeed, magic because in a little while, he felt
wonderful again. He was again eight feet tall in a lovely room,
feeling cheerful and silly, and happy and full of good spirits.
And again the same thing happened. Again he slept. And
again he awakened feeling sick. And again the old man offered
the magic potion, and as the days passed and turned into

weeks, and the weeks into months, the little boy drank the magic potion in greater amounts and more and more often.

After a very long time had passed, one morning when the little boy awakened, he looked about blearily and saw that the room was empty. He thought, "Oh, I must, I must leave here. I don't like feeling eight feet tall and then feeling so sick. I must get away from here." And so he crept out of the cabin, and he hid in the woods. Presently, he heard the old man come back into the hut and stomp around. He heard him come out and call. He heard him beat the bushes looking for him, but the small boy trembled and hid himself. At last the old man swore an oath and gave up. He went back into the hut.

After a little while, when the boy heard him snoring, he got up and ran away. But still he was lost in the forest and didn't know how he would get out again. He was feeling very sad and very frightened and very tired and full of despair when he became aware that he smelled smoke. He looked about, and in the distance he saw a campfire, around the campfire he saw a circle of people. Timidly he approached and as he came closer and closer, still feeling afraid, but beginning to feel a little hope, he smelled something delicious cooking on the campfire. He crept nearer and nearer, but he was so weak that before he could reach them he fell and was too faint to get up again. And as he lay there, almost unconscious in the leaves, he felt someone lifting him up in strong arms and carrying him.

When at last he dared to open his eyes, he was propped up among a group of people who were circling the campfire. When they saw that he had opened his eyes, they greeted him and asked his name. When he told them his name, they each said their names around the circle, and then they gave him a little cup filled with a delicious stew. At first he was afraid it was another magic potion and hesitated to eat it. But they said, "No, this is not a magic potion. This is good, healthful, nourishing food. Eat it without fear." So at last he did, and presently he could feel the strength coming back into his body. He stayed with these friendly people until his strength returned and he felt himself growing taller and strong.

Then one spring day, again he wished to leave the forest. And it came to pass that several of the people around the campfire decided to leave the forest together so the little boy went with them. His heart felt light and full of hope, because he was finding his way out of the forest. They had a map, and each day they drew closer to the edge of the dense forest until one day, they emerged into full sunlight, and the little boy's heart jumped with joy and hope as he looked about him.

But, they said to him, "We are not yet in the clear, for before us there is a very high and fierce mountain which we have to climb." And sure enough, there, ahead, was a huge barrier mountain. And his heart sank for he could not see how he could possibly have the strength or the skill to climb the mountain. But his friends said, "Watch us. Do what we do and you will make it. The first rule is not to look up and not to look back. The second rule is to find each handhold in turn on the face of the mountain, hand over hand, one foot after the other, and you will reach the top."

And so he started. It was slow and it was difficult and sometimes he thought his strength was not great enough and he would have to let go and fall back. But then he remembered not to look up ahead, and not to look back, but simply to look at each handhold in turn and each foothold, one after the other, until one day, he found himself gloriously at the top. As he looked out from the top of the mountain, he saw spread out below, a beautiful plain. There were gardens, there was a fine city teeming with happy, busy, active people, and he thought, "Oh, I must hurry to get there because then I will have returned to the world that I seek."

But with dismay he looked down and he saw that just as he had climbed the difficult climb up the mountain, now he must find his way down the other side, hand over hand and foot after foot. Then he said to himself with resolve, "It will be easier going down the mountain back to my world than it was climbing the mountain, for I will remember not to look ahead and not to look back, but to find each handhold, and each foothold, one after the other, and if I keep steady on, I will make it." And so he started down, remembering not to look back and not to look ahead, but steadily one foot after the other, one hand after the other, carefully, firmly planting each foot, firmly, carefully finding each handhold and he began to sing a little song as he climbed down the other side of the mountain to rejoin the world. And the song had a rhythm to it that went with his handhold and his foothold and it had a grace and a rhythm that increased in happiness and strength the nearer he approached the beautiful plain above which rose the fine city and the welcoming world. When he reached the bottom, he turned to look at the city spread out there in the sparkling light. He saw the people and the gardens, and then he ran forward with a shout of joy and happiness that at last he had found his way back from the forest.

Rick stayed in treatment for about 16 months. He continued attending AA meetings, he made a friend of his sponsor, and gradually joined a new circle of friends whom he found to be genuinely warm and supportive. He began to date women whom he met there, and had several love affairs in succession. His level of self-esteem rose steadily. He enrolled in a technical school to train to be an auto mechanic. He regularly attended AA meetings and eventually became a sponsor himself. His mother and father welcomed him back into his family and arranged for him to see his children with them. Even his brother and sisters became less hostile.

During the course of treatment, I told variations of "The Boy Who Lost His Way" from time to time. When eventually we spaced out our regular sessions, he came in at three- to four-month intervals, which we gradually spaced out to once a year. Now he no longer needs to come in.

18

The Little Elephant Who Didn't Know How to Cry

(A Story for a Client With Borderline Personality Disorder)

Jackie came swaggering into my office, her chin elevated, her shoulders squared, exuding an aura of defiance. She plunked herself down on the sofa, crossed her legs, bounced her foot, drummed her fingers, made spastic facial grimaces, and studiously avoided making eye contact. I remained silent. She began to giggle and to escalate her agitation. I waited. She bounced around on the sofa.

I said, "Do you think you are crazy?" She instantly stopped all movement, and looked at me for the first time. Then I saw the beginning of a sly smile. I added, "Because you are acting as if you want me to think you are crazy." She shrugged. I continued, "It is a choice, you know. You can opt for being crazy or you can choose to be sane. Even the inmates of mental institutions admit this when they are released, if you ask them." That was the beginning.

She told me about her father, whom she described as paranoid, and her mother, described as a borderline schizophrenic. Her own life was hemmed in by distrust and suspicion . . . angry, isolated, depraved by alcohol, drugs, and prostitution. Living alone, she accepted only nighttime jobs, so as to avoid human contact as much as possible. Her present job was as night attendant in an institution for "exceptional" children. She felt fiercely protective of them against the authority figures of the institution. Among the many things she spoke about was that she was so tough that even as a very little child they couldn't make her cry! She never cried!

*Jackie responded quickly to hypnosis and developed som-
nambulistic trance readily. Gradually, after she had tested me
repeatedly,* she began to trust me. After about 15 sessions,
which were focused primarily on creating rapport and trust
between us, the following story told itself.*

O nce upon a time there was a little elephant who got separated from her family when she was so little that she
couldn't remember them at all. The little elephant was adopt-
ed by a pair of outlaw elephants that did not belong to any
family and these outlaw elephants were very fierce and very
strong and very angry and sometimes afraid. But they didn't
have any fun. They didn't know how to have fun and they
never felt sad. So the little elephant grew ... knowing how
to be angry and to be afraid enough to protect herself, but
she didn't learn how to play or have fun, and she never learned
how to cry. And the little elephant didn't miss having fun or
crying because she had never experienced either one.

One day as she was ambling along in the sunshine, nibbling
on tender tree buds, smelling the rich jungle, and feeling the
gentle wind tickle her ears, the little elephant saw in the
distance a large herd of elephants. She had never seen such
a sight before, so she crept carefully through the long grass,

---

*Once she arrived without an appointment, high on cocaine, and began
to create an uproar in the waiting room. I led her into an empty treatment
room, calmly told her to lie down and sleep, and said I would return in an
hour. Quite docilely she did as she was told. When I returned, she was just
waking up.

keeping her eyes fixed on the herd, ready to run at an instant's alarm, every bristly hair on her hide standing straight up with fear. But still, curiosity overcame her fear and she kept creeping closer and closer soundlessly to watch the family of elephants. And she saw the strangest things happen. She saw them romping and pushing and raising their trunks making funny chortling noises. She saw them splashing in the stream, and spraying each other with water through their trunks, and they seemed not to be afraid and not to be angry. They seemed to be doing something else altogether strange and new. The little elephant watched with fascination, ready to turn and run at a moment's notice, but still so fascinated that she stayed rooted to the spot to watch them.

Suddenly there was a strange noise and the little elephant sensed that there was danger near. Instantly she got herself prepared with a large surge of anger and fear to protect herself, and as she waved her trunk in all directions to scent what danger threatened, she saw an amazing thing. The family of elephants had formed a circle and all of them were standing shoulder to shoulder with their tails pointing to the center of the circle and their long gray trunks facing out. The leader of the elephants, a great big bull elephant, was trumpeting orders in an ear-splitting screeching bellow. And so they closed ranks and stood still. All the big elephants stood in a circle facing out, and then the little elephant noticed with surprise and wonder that there were dozens of little elephants who were inside the circle being protected by the full-grown adults. And she watched with astonishment that they would do such a thing.

Then she scented the smell of a lion in the air! She trembled and looked about for a place to hide. Suddenly without warning she felt herself nudged from behind and pushed forcibly. She turned to fight fiercely, but there stood a huge, grumbling, gray elephant behind her who said in a deep voice, "Hurry, hurry, what is wrong with you? Get in the middle right away. Didn't you hear the warning?" And the little elephant said, "But I don't belong." And the big elephant looked down at her and said, "Nonsense, you are one of us. I recognize you. Get in the middle. Get in the center right away."

The little elephant hesitated, shuffling her feet, then decided to obey instead of running away, and she went into the center with all the other little elephants. She looked around and although she was still trembling with fear could scarcely believe what was happening, she still had the strangest feeling in her chest. She felt as though her chest were swelling up . . . and it felt very good to be there.

When the danger had passed, the elephants broke their circle and they began to nudge and urge the young ones into a line. The little elephant saw that the big bull elephant led the line, and the next elephant took the tail of the leader elephant with its trunk and another elephant came up and took that elephant's tail in its trunk, and another took that elephant's tail and so they formed a long line with each elephant holding the tail of the elephant in front in its trunk and they began their journey. The little elephant stayed with the herd and watched and tried to learn from them. But when they all played and pushed and splashed each other, she stood aside and didn't know how to join in, even though the others called her and pushed her and tried to get her to have fun with them. When they called and pushed she would bristle with fear and anger and try to frighten them away because she didn't know how to play.

One day, one of the big elephants observed how the little elephant would not play and also noticed that when she hurt herself, she didn't cry. And that elephant called a conference with the other wise elephants. They put their trunks together and they thought of what to do. And so they made a plan. They called the little elephant over and they said, "You are getting bigger now and it is time that you join in the family world. So we're going to put you in charge of these six very small newborn elephants, and you will be responsible for them. They will be your charges and you must take care of them." The little elephant felt very good about that. Also, she knew how to protect them because she had learned very well how to be angry and fierce, and also how to be afraid so she would know when to be angry and fierce. And so she rounded them up and she taught them their manners and she saw that they were safe. Day after day passed, and the little elephants grew to love her very much. Wherever she went, they would follow after. If she turned away, they would call to her and when she was near they would snuggle up to her for warmth and affection. The little elephant found that she felt very good every day. She felt better and better. The days passed uneventfully and peacefully. She felt safe, and no longer needed to be afraid so often or to be angry at all.

One day as she and her six little elephants wandered down a shady lane into the jungle, there was a sudden noise, and without warning, a huge lion jumped out at them, grabbed the last little baby elephant, and in the flash of an eye, made off with it before the little elephant could sound a warning or protect it. With a heavy heart, she took the five little elephants back to the herd, went up to the leader bull elephant, and sadly told what had happened. The bull elephant looked down at her, and he saw that the little elephant had water in her eyes. She felt the water in her eyes, and felt the water running down all along the inside of her long trunk. She looked up at the big elephant and asked, "What is happening?" And the big elephant said, "You are crying." The little elephant felt her tears, and the big elephant said, "You have just experienced compassion and sadness." The little elephant sat down, experiencing her sadness and her compassion.

After that, she began to recognize that she was feeling love for her five little elephants, and they for her. And with her feelings of love and her tears, she began to learn to play with them, and to laugh, and to spray water, and push and tumble. And so she grew up . . . a happy elephant with her family . . . protected, safe, able to be fierce and angry, able to be afraid, but also able to cry tears and to love.

Jackie came in the next session saying, "What the hell is this with elephants? I keep dreaming about elephants. I think about elephants all the time. I'm sick of elephants." But changes began to appear. She changed jobs, but chose another nighttime assignment in the admissions department of a large hospital, where she had more contact with people. She visited her parents. She started a friendship with another woman which lasted some months, albeit stormily. Gradually, she made friends, stopped abusing drugs, and cut down on alcohol, as we continued hypnotherapy. She then enrolled in a training school for radio broadcasting. She proved to have a very good voice and enunciation, as well as an aptitude for creating advertising announcements. She formed an ongoing relationship with a lover, and seemed quite happy. When she landed a job as a radio announcer in a small nearby town, she terminated therapy.

19
Transformation

(A Story Told as Part of the
Termination Process
of Treatment)

When the time comes to terminate a client's treatment, I often use the following story as a bridge to facilitate the crossing over into separation and individuation. I may vary the telling somewhat for each client's particular frame of reference, but basically it is this story as I tell it here.

O nce upon a time, deep in a quiet, dark forest, in the heart of a quiet, dark forest, stood a tree. And on one of its uppermost branches there hung a curious object. It resembled a little brown silken pouch, and it hung on the underside of a high branch deep in the quiet, dark forest. The little silk pouch hung there through a long, long winter. Inside the pouch slept a quiet creature . . . sleeping, sleeping a quiet, deep sleep, its little body curled up, motionless. But all through the cold winter, warm inside its silken pouch, the little body kept growing . . . so slowly you couldn't be sure, but growing it was, and as it grew bigger and bigger, the silken pouch fit more and more snugly, and held the little creature more tightly, but still the little body kept growing and growing until one spring day, it had grown so big that the silken pouch gently began to tear. As it tore, a larger and larger opening appeared in its side, until one day the pouch opened from one end to the other. The little creature stirred and felt its new space. Then cautiously, trembling in all its fragile body, it pushed its head outside the pouch. It couldn't see very much because the forest was still quite dark and its eyes were still only partly open. It could hear murmurings, and it could see soft, vague shapes, it could smell a wonderful and tantalizing fragrance. And so, trembling, it dared to emerge yet farther and farther from within its soft, silken prison. And when at last it crept free of the pouch, it stood on shaky legs, all wet and skinny and very, very unsure of itself.

In the sky, over the trees in the forest, the sun shone brightly and the golden light filtered down through the leaves in a patchwork of shapes and patterns. There just ahead, with ever strengthening eyesight, it saw a bright shape on the bough and, lured by the shining, beautiful color, the little creature cautiously crept forward inch by inch, stopping at every small step to look about fearfully. And at last, entirely free of the little brown pouch, it moved right into the golden shape. There it felt the warmth, the warmth of the color, almost heard the vibrating sound of the golden color, and the fragrance it smelled was also golden. As the warmth spread over its body, it felt energy tingling and beginning to surge. Steadily it began to feel its strength and it stood up ever straighter, lifting its head. Then it discovered wondrous long feelers at the top of its head that could sense all around it the new world of the forest. Its heart began to swell with a feeling, and a sense almost like love, almost like power, almost like strength, almost like joy.

And as it grew warmer and warmer in the golden shape that surrounded it, it began to unfold from its body a wonderful, wonderful pair of translucent wings that kept spreading wider and wider. And on the wings there emerged a fantastic pattern of glorious color and shape and design, and the little creature trembled as it allowed its wings to flutter gently in the sunlight. As they dried, they became ever more powerful until at last the little creature began rhythmically as in a dance, it began rhythmically raising and lowering its two beautiful wings. Ever more quickly, ever more powerfully, the marvelous wings beat the air until, with a surging leap into space, the little creature soared upwards higher and higher until it was flying, gliding, dipping, held up by the air, propelled forward by the strength of its wings, sailing in a graceful dance high above the forest . . . free, beautiful, and winging its own way into the welcoming world.

My hope, as I bring these stories to a close, is that those of you who have not as yet ventured on this particular journey will trust the strength of your wings and take flight.

Listen carefully now with the "third ear," you might hear the sound of wings . . .

New England Institute For NLP
RFD #3, Pratt Corner Rd.
Amherst, MA 01002-9805
(413) 259-1248
Towards Greater Excellence